COMPLETE
detox
WORKBOOK

COMPLETE
detox
WORKBOOK

2-day, 9-day and 30-day makeovers to cleanse and revitalize your life

Dr Christina Scott-Moncrieff
MB ChB MFHom

COLLINS & BROWN

This edition published in the United Kingdom in 2015

Collins & Brown

1 Gower Street

London

WC1E 6HD

An imprint of Pavilion Books Company Ltd

Distributed in the United States and Canada by Sterling Publishing Co, 387 Park Avenue South,
New York, NY 10016-8810, USA

ISBN 978-1-91023-135-7

A CIP catalogue record for this book is available from the British Library.

10 9 8 7 6 5 4 3 2 1

Reproduction by Colourdepth Ltd, UK

Printed and bound by Times Offset (M) SDN BHD, Malaysia

This book can be ordered direct from the publisher at www.pavilionbooks.com

Front cover photography: Shutterstock

Photography on pages 5, 9, 23, 29, 45, 46, 59, 71, 73, 104, 105, 109, 111, 112 by Sian Irvine

SAFETY NOTE

The information in this book is not intended as a substitute for medical advice.
Any person suffering from conditions requiring medical attention, or who has
symptoms that concern them, should consult a qualified medical practitioner.

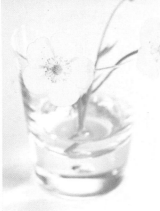

contents

Introduction

Detox is for everyone. Everyone, that is, who longs to have an abundance of physical energy, to be mentally calm and in control and to have the freedom of choice that comes from feeling really well.

Detox is about improving your quality of life, not just for now, but also for the future; not just physically, but also mentally and emotionally. Every year statistics show that people are living longer. With detox it is possible to improve the quality of these extra years.

Why do we feel less than 100 per cent so often? Why do we seem to be short of energy and notice so many niggling aches and pains or tolerate symptoms that are more intrusive? Feeling 'out of control' or 'tired all the time' may not be symptoms that appear in many medical textbooks, but they are heard with increasing frequency in the consulting rooms of every doctor and healthcare professional.

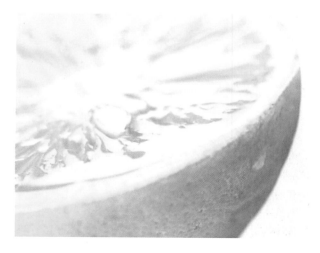

HOW TOXINS CAN AFFECT OUR HEALTH

The answer lies in 'toxins'. This word is used to describe the chemicals in the body that have not been made harmless, or 'detoxed'. Some of these chemicals are the result of our living in an increasingly polluted world, and some are caused by poor diets that do not supply the body with the nutrients it needs to perform the usual detox functions effectively. These toxins can affect our ability to think properly; they can produce physical symptoms such as exhaustion or headaches; and create emotional turmoil such as anger and frustration, or feelings of misery and hopelessness.

EVERYONE CAN BENEFIT FROM DETOX

You do not have to put up with all this. Detox gives you the opportunity to take a grip on your health and the way you feel, and everyone who decides to make the effort can benefit at least a little but often to a surprisingly great extent. What is more, you can choose between making a major effort and seeing rapid improvements or introducing changes gradually to fit a busy life. If this gradual approach is all that is possible, the resulting improvement may occur so slowly that it is barely noticeable, but progress can be charted by noting the scores achieved when answering the symptoms questionnaire on pp. 22–23 of the book. It is often helpful to repeat this exercise every few months.

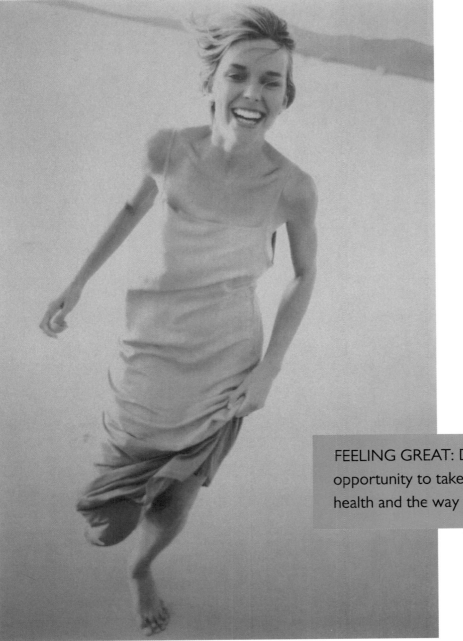

FEELING GREAT: Detox provides the opportunity to take a grip on your health and the way you feel.

THE DETOX PROGRAMME

Following a detox programme reduces the amount of toxins entering your body and helps your body to deal with them better by improving nutrition and enhancing the removal of unwanted waste. This book provides a choice between programmes that allow you to work as usual and more intensive programmes that require a short retreat from the world. It also guides you towards the lo-tox lifestyle that will help you to go on feeling fit and energetic. If you have any medical condition or symptoms that you have not discussed with your doctor, you should obtain advice before starting a programme.

PART ONE

What is detox and who needs it?

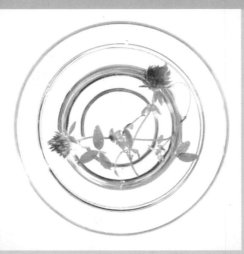

Health is more than the absence of disease – you need to feel well.

What is **detox?**

Every day most of us encounter natural chemicals that can cause damage or irritation to the body. By detoxing you can help your system to deal with these toxins and maintain your health and well-being.

The world is not a friendly place. Every day we encounter unfriendly chemicals and other toxic substances that can cause damage or irritation to our bodies unless they are changed by being 'detoxified' into safer substances. Every cell in the body contributes to this 'detox' process, which is essentially the disposal of waste.

Rubbish left in the street or an overflowing sewer can become health hazards. In the same way, when our detox systems cannot cope, for whatever reason, a backlog of unwanted waste builds up in our bodies, which, at the very least, leaves us feeling below par but can cause illness.

NATURALLY OCCURRING TOXINS

As part of the evolutionary process, our bodies have learned to defend themselves from naturally occurring toxins by changing them into safer substances and getting rid of them as soon as possible. They are discharged in stools, mucus and bile; in urine, sweat and tears; and even in our hair and nails.

Natural toxins can be produced within the body when, for example, it is fighting infection, dealing with the biochemical after-effects of stress or simply performing routine repair and maintenance. The word biochemistry means the chemistry of life. In order to maintain life and health, our bodies continually monitor internal biochemical processes and deal with any harmful chemicals that arise.

Natural toxins also occur in the environment. For example, many plants produce toxic substances to protect themselves against predators. Although we have learned to avoid the highly poisonous plants that would overwhelm our systems, many of the everyday plants that we eat contain substances that can kill small pests such as caterpillars. Provided our detox systems are working properly, we are able to detoxify these substances with ease.

SO WHY CAN'T WE ALWAYS DETOX EFFECTIVELY?

One common reason why our bodies become overwhelmed with toxins is that our diets are often poor, lacking many vital nutrients. You may find this surprising when you look around a supermarket that contains several thousand different food stuffs, but it is true.

In the West we have sacrificed food quality for convenience, and many packaged foods have had vital nutrients removed. This may be done intentionally to prolong shelf life or for other reasons, including public demand. For example, most people eat white bread and rolls, even though 90 per cent of the magnesium, a mineral essential to effective detoxing, has been milled

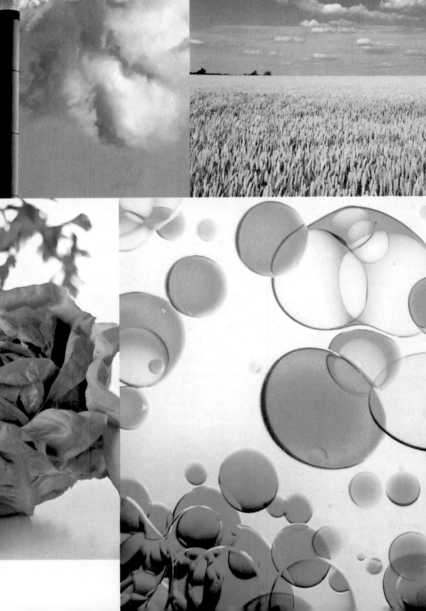

Detoxing and a good diet can help your body to cope with the build up of harmful toxins in the body caused by air pollution, pesticides and fungicides.

out of it. Nor can we blame the food industry entirely for losses from prolonged storage times: when shops do sell really fresh fruit and vegetables, vital vitamins can be lost when we shop only once a week and keep our food for several days in the fridge.

As a result of these changes, some vital nutrients have been lost, resulting in our detox systems becoming less effective at detoxing all the unfriendly chemicals entering our bodies. This is a little like employing refuse collectors to go around the town emptying the dustbins, but equipping them with handcarts instead of automatically loading lorries. Even if they were able to cope, their efforts would hardly be very efficient.

WHEN THE **DETOX SYSTEMS** CAN'T COPE…

Unchanged, or only partially changed, toxins are left to roam through the body, causing damage and a decline in the feeling of 'wellness' that we usually take for granted. Symptoms can vary widely from person to person, but the most common problem is constant tiredness.

Doctors working in environmental medicine believe that improving diet quality, taking measures to reduce stress and avoiding man-made chemicals whenever possible can help our body's detox system and enhance general health and well-being.

POLLUTION IS AN ADDED PROBLEM

Since the middle of the twentieth century we have been increasingly exposed to the vast numbers of new substances that have been produced by the chemical industry, often, but not always, for the best of reasons. They can enter the body by being eaten, inhaled or absorbed through the skin. However, few of them have a useful function once inside the body, and they have to be made safe by our detox systems. Doctors who specialize in environmental medicine sometimes use the term 'total load' to describe the burden imposed by being exposed to so many toxins.

Today, many of the foods we eat contain minute amounts of man-made pesticides, fungicides and herbicides. Use of these chemicals is tightly controlled in most countries, but the rules are still sometimes broken. Unfortunately, only a small proportion of agricultural produce is tested for the presence of these chemicals, but when it is, the results sometimes reveal levels of contamination that give cause for concern. In addition, even crops that are grown organically can be contaminated by chemical sprays being applied many miles away.

In the past 50 years, additional airborne pollution has increased the introduction of toxins into our bodies through our lungs. This has been the result of our increasing use of cars; homes and offices being maintained at comfortable temperatures; chemical treatment for woodworm and for dry or wet rot; perfumes and deodorants, and chemicals that help us to keep our clothes and buildings clean with the minimum of effort. Cigarette smoke is a clear source of inhaled toxins, but many other less obvious chemicals that we cannot smell find their way into our bodies as we breathe. They all add to the total load.

Our use of medicines is another area of concern, as most of them need to be detoxed by the liver.

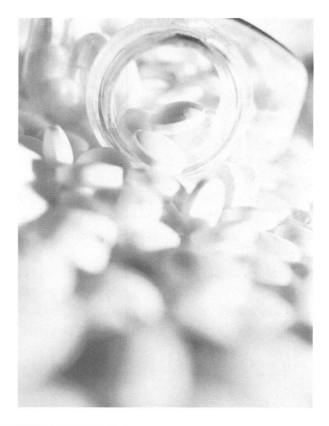

Although our skin is waterproof and acts as a barrier to keep out unwanted watery substances, it cannot prevent the absorption of any chemical that dissolves in fat or oil. Many recently created chemicals can enter our bodies in this way, as can the constituents of cosmetics and other products that are marketed for skin care.

Another problem arises with our greater use of medicines, as these usually have to be detoxed in the liver. There are also concerns about the medication routinely given to intensively reared animals. Although the marketing of meat from these animals is tightly controlled, regulations are difficult to police, and it is likely that medicine residues creep into the food chain. As contamination of the oceans and fresh water occurs, toxic chemicals can also enter the food chain in fish.

FOOD **ADDITIVES**

Almost every bought food that has been pre-cooked, pre-packed or processed in any way contains food additives such as preservatives, colouring agents, thickeners and flavour enhancers. It has been estimated that by the time children reach the age of 18 they will have eaten their own body weight in food additives.

Many of these substances are added for reasons of safety, to avoid spoilage and to prolong shelf life. Unfortunately, the resulting convenience and extended shelf life are mixed blessings, as all of these chemicals have to be processed by the body.

This uses vital energy and nutrients, and potentially clogs up the detox system when it could be working on other substances that are less avoidable. Furthermore, although food additives (and the pesticides, fungicides and herbicides that are used in farming and food storage) have been individually tested for safety, very little research has been performed to test their safety when they are mixed together or consumed over a long time. Food additives have been linked to asthma, rashes and, in children, hyperactivity.

How toxic is **your lifestyle?**

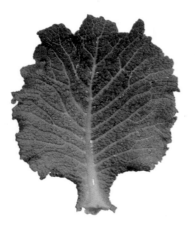

Work through this checklist of lifestyle choices that could be adding to the amount of toxins your body has to deal with. How many have you answered 'yes' to?

LESS THAN 10: Your lifestyle is already very healthy, and detox should be easy for you.

BETWEEN 11 AND 20: You should be able to help reduce the 'total load' (p. 12) without too much effort.

MORE THAN 21: You have some way to go, but do not become alarmed, as you are certainly not alone. Just reading this questionnaire should help you to become more aware of the areas in your life that could be contributing to your total load.

Whatever your score, you will find many useful suggestions in Part Two of this book to help you implement positive changes.

FOOD AND DRINK

Do you eat or drink the following frequently?

❑ Tea or coffee

❑ Sodas or other fizzy drinks

❑ Convenience or processed meals or foods

❑ White bread, pasta, rice and other grains

❑ Snack foods such as crisps or sweets

❑ Foods containing artificial sweeteners (often in 'diet foods')

❑ Smoked foods (such as bacon, fish, cheese and cooked meats)

❑ Barbecued food

❑ Non-organic fruit (without washing and peeling first)

❑ Non-organic green vegetables (without removing outer leaves)

❑ Non-organic root vegetables (without scrubbing and peeling)

❑ Processed meats (sausages, burgers, pies, etc.)

❑ Fried foods

❑ Salt (including sea salt) added both during cooking and on your plate

❑ More alcohol than is recommended as the safe intake (two units a day for women and three for men.)

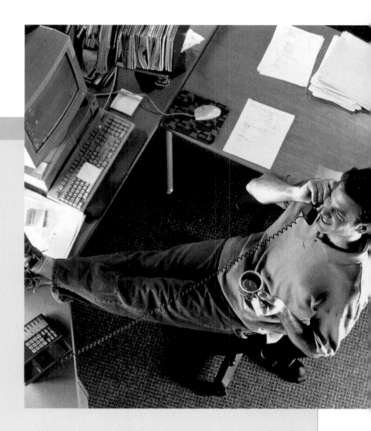

ENVIRONMENT

Answer these questions about your surroundings.

❏ Do you live in a city or within a mile of a major road?

❏ Do you live under a busy flight path?

❏ Do you often walk or run along busy roads?

❏ Do you live near fields that are regularly sprayed?

❏ Do you often swim in a pool containing chlorinated water?

❏ Do you use a mobile phone?

❏ Does your house have cavity wall insulation?

❏ Is your home double glazed?

❏ Do you have central heating or air conditioning?

❏ Have you recently had your house treated for woodworm or rot or put in new timber?

❏ Have you recently bought soft furnishings, especially those with 'stain resistant' finishes?

❏ Do you have your clothes dry-cleaned regularly?

❏ Have you recently laid a new carpet or vinyl flooring?

❏ Do you have much chipboard, fibreboard, plywood or MDF in your house?

❏ Is your plumbing more than 20 years old?

❏ Is the paintwork in your house very old or have you recently repainted?

❏ Do you use synthetic air fresheners?

❏ Do you use pesticides in your house or garden?

❏ Do you use large amounts of bleach, detergent, household cleaners or disinfectant?

❏ Do you live near a power station or within half a mile of high-voltage overhead power cables?

❏ Do you work with a computer?

❏ Do you smoke?

❏ Do you live in an area where the underlying rock is granite, shale or sedimentary rock?

❏ Do you cook or heat your house with gas-powered appliances?

Decline and **recovery**

Our decline in health usually comes on slowly and imperceptibly. We often put down feeling less than perfect to 'stress' or 'getting older', when in fact these mild symptoms are signs that our detox systems are beginning to feel the strain.

Our natural ability to detox helps us to live with chemicals that we really ought to avoid. To do this, a chain of events takes place in which there are three successive stages to the way that the body reacts to toxins: initial reaction, adaptation and exhaustion.

A good example is smoking. Few people really enjoy their first cigarette and most have an initial reaction in which they either feel sick or have a rapid bowel action. Despite this, some people go on smoking and become able to tolerate 20, 40 or even 80 cigarettes a day without developing unpleasant symptoms. This is because their bodies have learned to cope with, or adapt to, the toxic chemicals. This phenomenon is also known as 'masking', but its effects can be lost. For example, if a heavy smoker quits but smokes a cigarette a few years later, the chances are it will be very unpleasant. People who detox from caffeine often develop palpitations or insomnia when they later start to drink coffee again.

The main problem with masking, however, is its cost in terms of using up energy and nutrients. Once we become 'masked' to a chemical that provides pleasant feelings, such as relaxation from nicotine or extra energy from caffeine, we tend to become 'addicted' and indulge more frequently. As a result, there is less energy and fewer nutrients to deal with toxins that we cannot avoid, such as those produced naturally within our bodies (see pp. 18–19).

This leads to the exhaustion stage, which develops gradually as the body loses its reserves and can no longer adapt sufficiently to avoid symptoms. The first signs include loss of energy, digestive disturbances, a weakened immune system and raised blood pressure. Eventually, serious diseases may develop. Smokers are prone to heart disease, lung cancer and other respiratory diseases; drinkers may develop liver diseases, and those who eat too much refined sugar can develop late-onset diabetes with all its complications.

DETOX AND RECOVER

Although detoxing appears to be a modern idea, fasting and dietary changes have been used for many centuries to restore health. They are an essential part of Ayurvedic medicine, and there are many references to them in the Bible, the Koran and early Greek writings. More recently, they have been a part of naturopathic medical practice. In the West, however, many conventional medical practitioners lost their belief that such measures could help to prevent illness when powerful modern drugs became available.

Recent advances in biochemical knowledge are giving scientific respectability to the view that some of the chronic illnesses of older age can be postponed,

DETOX WORKS: It restores energy levels, improves digestion and strengthens resistance to infection.

or even avoided, by the adoption of a healthy lifestyle. There are now many doctors and therapists whose patients have had their health restored by reducing their exposure to chemicals and increasing their supply of nutrients. This is the basis of detoxing, which can be the first step to a healthy future.

How does **detox occur?**

Some people inherit better detox systems than others, and younger people tend to have more efficient systems than older people. But a poor diet and exposure to toxic chemicals can negate these natural advantages.

Occasionally, damage from chemical exposure is permanent, which obviously limits our ability to detox, but this is unlikely to be a problem in the absence of other illness, in which case professional advice is essential. The good news is that, for most of us whose lifestyle has been less than perfect, the body's capacity for boosting our detox system and recovering is often amazingly good. So how do our bodies deal with these toxins?

THE DIGESTIVE SYSTEM

A healthy digestive system is one of the first lines of defence. It breaks down food to release nutrients, regulates what the body absorbs and discharges any waste that is left over. Useful bacteria living in the large intestine produce additional waste that also needs to be discharged in the stool. Effective elimination of waste from the bowel is essential, as it is one of the routes the liver uses to discharge unwanted toxins from our bodies.

THE LIVER

Although every cell in our body has the ability to take up harmful chemicals and detoxify them, the major organ of detox is the liver. Each minute it receives about three pints of blood for cleansing. Most of the food that we eat is taken in the blood straight from the intestine to the liver for detox, and only then is it released for circulation to the rest of the body.

The liver removes dead or abnormal cells, yeasts, bacteria, viruses, parasites, incompletely digested or abnormal proteins, artificial chemicals and any other

SYMPTOMS OF LIVER **OVERLOAD**

- Poor digestion, bloating, nausea, constipation or other bowel irregularity.
- Unpleasant mood changes, depression, poor concentration and forgetfulness.
- Onset or worsening of allergic conditions such as hay fever, skin rashes and asthma.
- Headaches.
- Raised blood pressure and/or fluid retention.
- Poorly controlled levels of sugar in the blood, causing fatigue, dizziness, sugar craving or light-headedness.
- Decreased tolerance of fatty foods or alcohol.
- Excessive sweating and unpleasant body odour.

dangerous or foreign particles. Hormones are taken out of the circulation once they have completed their functions, and the dangerous ammonia that is formed when aged proteins are broken down is mopped up by our liver, which converts it to urea and sends it off to be discharged in urine.

Unfortunately, the liver is often the first organ to suffer when our detox systems become overwhelmed. Not only can it no longer perform its detox tasks, but its numerous other functions also suffer, causing many different symptoms (see box, left).

THE SKIN

The skin, the largest organ of our bodies, has an important role in detox. Sweat contains urea and a number of other waste products, some of which are eliminated only through the skin. In recent years some doctors have been recommending treatments such as saunas and exercise to increase the production of sweat and aid the removal of a number of toxic chemicals from the body. As detox programmes progress, it is not unusual to notice that your skin begins to 'glow' and to look younger and less wrinkled.

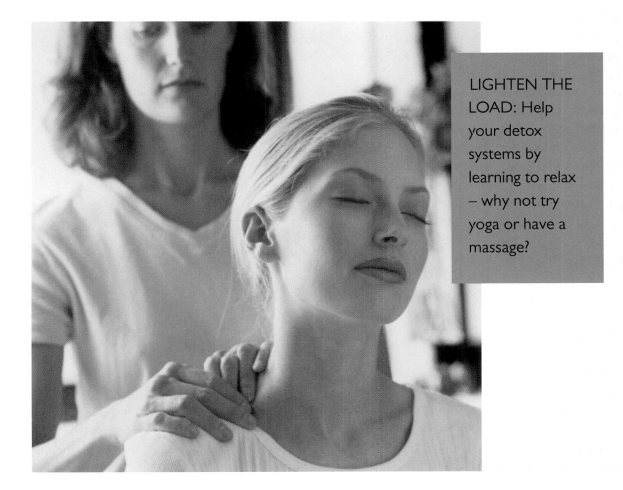

LIGHTEN THE LOAD: Help your detox systems by learning to relax – why not try yoga or have a massage?

THE KIDNEYS

The kidneys filter the blood and remove a number of the toxins, including urea (see pp. 18–19), which the liver has changed so that they dissolve in water. Our kidneys work best when we drink plenty of water, especially during a detox programme when the body is being given the opportunity of cleansing itself (see box, right).

WHAT CAN A DETOX PROGRAMME ACHIEVE?

A detox programme is designed to enhance your body's own natural detoxing ability. As a result:

You will feel better without a backlog of unchanged or partially changed toxins causing symptoms. Your body will work more efficiently, as it will have a steady supply of all the nutrients it needs and fewer or no foods that contain 'empty calories' (see p. 39). 'Empty-calorie' foods provide energy, but are bereft of nutrients to help the energy systems of the body. In processing these foods the body uses minerals and vitamins that might be better employed elsewhere.

Any addictions will be reduced or even cured. You will feel more in control, as you will no longer be driven by your need for a cigarette, a coffee, a bar of chocolate or whatever you cannot imagine living without (see also food intolerance, p. 88; and addictive chemicals, p. 41).

Your body will not be wasting energy on dealing with foreign chemicals that it does not need. As a result, you will feel less tired and even regain extra energy that you had lost, which is a bonus for work or recreation.

Once the body's internal biochemistry regains a balance, you will be less prone to episodes of low blood sugar, which make you feel shaky, hungry and irritable.

Your immune system will be strengthened so that you should be better able to fight off infections, and you may also reduce the risk of developing a cancer.

Weight control should be easier, whether you are overweight or underweight.

Many women find cellulite disappears.

10 REASONS TO DRINK **MORE WATER**

Drink at least six to eight glasses of water each day, and more in warm weather or if you are taking exercise or sweating for any other reason. Alcohol and drinks that contain caffeine, such as tea, coffee and cola, do not count as the same volume of water, because they increase the loss of water from the body in urine. This leaves the body dehydrated. But you can flavour water with slices of organic lemon or lime or with their juice if the fruit is not organic. Water helps to:

- Flush out your kidneys and liver, enabling them to remove unwanted substances.
- Keep energy levels up: a 2 per cent loss of water surrounding the cells of the body can lead to a loss of energy by up to 20 per cent.
- Reduce the risk of developing gallstones and kidney stones.
- Relieve constipation.
- Reduce the risk of developing headaches.
- Make your immune system work effectively.
- Keep your brain active: dehydration may contribute to memory loss and senility.
- Reduce feelings of hunger: try water as a snack!
- Keep your skin looking good and feeling soft.
- Control the temperature of the body and eliminate toxins by sweating.

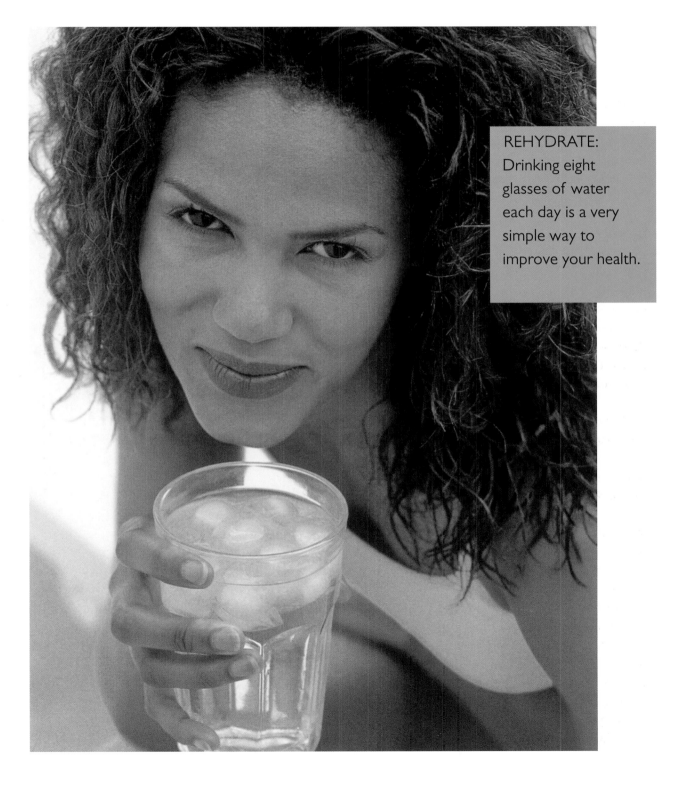

REHYDRATE:
Drinking eight
glasses of water
each day is a very
simple way to
improve your health.

Detox **questionnaire**

Take a little time to answer this questionnaire, as it will help you to assess your need to follow a detox programme. Score as follows: never = no points; rarely = 1 point; occasionally = 2 points; frequently = 3 points; all the time = 4 points.

Do you get any of these symptoms?

❑ Headaches or migraines	❑ A runny nose (but not a cold)	❑ Other rashes
❑ Disturbed sleep	❑ An itchy nose	❑ Hot flushes
❑ Watery or itchy eyes	❑ An itchy palate	❑ Excessive sweating
❑ Dark circles under your eyes	❑ A sore tongue	❑ Sweat with an unpleasant smell
❑ Itchy ears	❑ A furred tongue	❑ Irregular heartbeat
❑ Sneezing attacks	❑ Acne	❑ Rapid heartbeat
❑ A chronic cough	❑ Hives (nettle rash)	❑ Heartburn or indigestion
❑ Nausea or vomiting	❑ Feeling shaky and weak	❑ Being more tired than you would expect for your age and level of activity
❑ Diarrhoea	❑ Binge eating	
❑ Constipation	❑ Binge drinking or exceeding the safe drinking limit	❑ Feeling overactive or agitated without an immediate cause
❑ Bloated feeling	❑ Cravings for certain foods	
❑ Belching	❑ Compulsive eating	❑ Being restless and unable to settle
❑ Passing excessive or offensive wind	❑ Water retention	❑ Having problems with your memory
❑ Pain in joints	❑ Urinary frequency	
❑ Stiff joints	❑ Feeling very tired in the morning	❑ Feeling confused
❑ Aching or painful muscles		

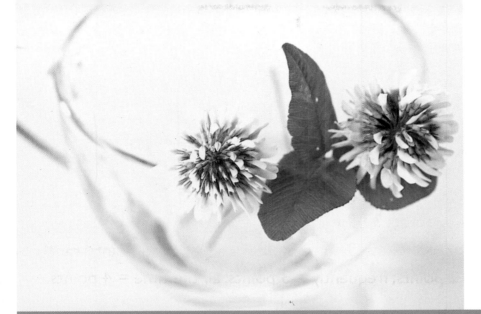

Do you get any of these symptoms?

- Being unable to understand new information or instructions
- Poor concentration
- Clumsiness
- Problems with your speech
- Having difficulty making decisions
- Unexplained feelings such as anxiety or fear
- Unprovoked anger, irritability or aggressiveness

- Depression
- Mood swings
- Sensitivity to light
- Sensitivity to noise

SCORE AS FOLLOWS:

rarely = 1

occasionally = 2

frequently = 3

all the time = 4

Finally, are you overweight?

Are you underweight?

Do you find difficulty in attaining or maintaining the correct weight for your height?

A 'yes' to any of these questions scores 3.

ADD UP YOUR TOTAL SCORE

WHAT IT MEANS

Check your total score. If you have:
- **LESS THAN 30:** This is excellent – a detox programme could help you to be symptom-free.
- **30–60:** Try to make time for a 30-Day Makeover or Detox in Nine Days programme and you will soon feel really good.
- **61–100:** You should soon notice the differences when you detox. To minimize withdrawal symptoms,

make sure that you detox from chemicals (pp. 34–43) before you start a programme.
- **MORE THAN 100:** Detox should make a real difference to the way you feel, but start gently. Try to reduce your exposure to chemicals as much as you can. Whatever your score, write it in your diary for future reference so that you can measure how much better you feel when you have detoxed.

What does **detox involve?**

Many people embarking on a detox programme feel as if they are venturing into the unknown. It is often helpful to have an idea of what to expect if you start a detox programme.

A detox programme simply means that you will be taking measures to reduce your exposure to man-made chemicals, ensuring that you are eating plenty of the nutrients your body needs to change existing toxins into safer substances and helping your body to expel them. It can also help to take measures to reduce stress in your life.

IS A DETOX PROGRAMME DIFFICULT?

This really depends on how much help your detox system needs to do its task effectively and how you want to approach the problem. Some people like to ease their way into a healthier lifestyle by taking several small steps. Others prefer to make a major change and get it over quickly.

One of the advantages of following the 30-Day Makeover programme is that by sticking to a restricted diet for four weeks, you will become accustomed to healthier food choices and you may be less tempted to return to old habits.

However, you might find it easier to detox in several short bursts, in which case you should plan a series of Weekend Energizers or a programme that involves short periods of detox every month or so, possibly coinciding with each change of season. Over time, you will achieve results that are just as good as if you had followed a longer or stricter detox programme. If

WHAT WILL DETOX **DO FOR ME?**

After detox most people find they have:

- Increased energy
- Better sleep
- Fewer mood swings
- Clearer thinking
- Fewer and shorter infections
- Less abdominal bloating
- Regular bowel movements
- Healthier skin
- Lessening of allergy symptoms

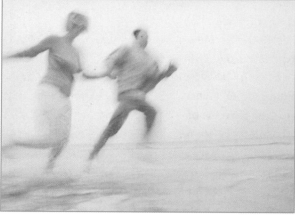

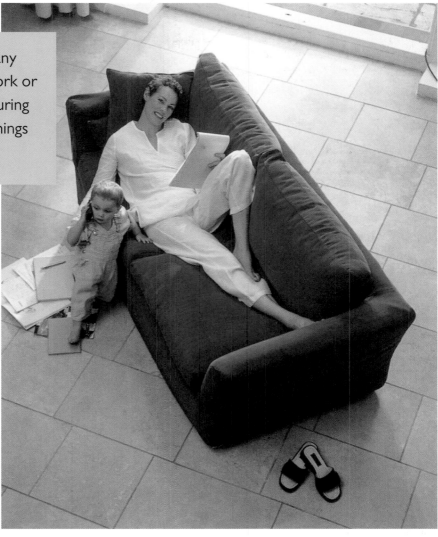

WORKING DETOX: Many people cannot give up work or domestic responsibility during a detox, but try to take things as gently as possible.

you are particularly impatient and can devote only a week or so to your first detox, then try the Detox in Nine Days programme. Be aware, however, that this is a strict regime, and if this is your first detox, you may experience quite severe withdrawal symptoms or side effects.

HOW WILL I FEEL?

Your tongue may become furred up, and your breath and sweat may smell unpleasant. You may feel nauseous and have headaches and general aches and pains in your muscles. Some people experience old symptoms such as catarrh, or they become irritable and depressed. These symptoms are generally worst in the first few days and are best thought of as a cleansing crisis, after which you will probably begin to feel calmer and more energetic as your body cleanses out unwanted rubbish. In general, we accumulate toxins over time, and the cleansing crises, if they occur, become less marked each time you follow a detox programme. There are measures you can take to help reduce the severity of many of these withdrawal symptoms (see pp. 82–85).

CAN I GO ON SMOKING?

If you are a smoker you probably have a greater need to detox than a non-smoker, and stopping smoking is the best thing you can do to help your detox system (see p. 42). In general, non-smokers are healthier than smokers. Even if you feel you cannot give up completely, try to smoke as little as possible during

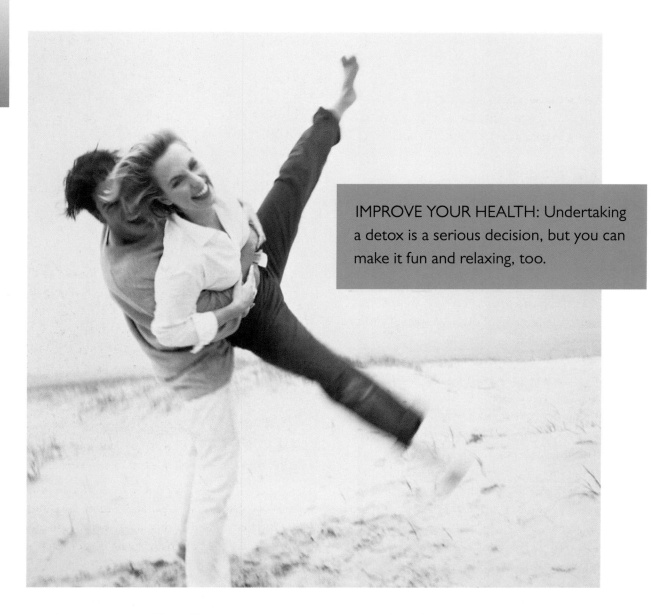

IMPROVE YOUR HEALTH: Undertaking a detox is a serious decision, but you can make it fun and relaxing, too.

your detox programme. You will probably feel so much better and less stressed as a result of the programme that the decision to give up smoking altogether will be much easier.

IS DETOXING COMPATIBLE WITH WORK?

This depends on which programme you decide to follow. The short, sharp mini-fasts and mono-diets are best followed at a time when you can take it easy and spoil yourself. If you wish to follow the fairly strict Detox in Nine Days regime, you should try to set aside a week in which you have a light schedule or, even better, are on holiday.

The 30-Day Makeover programme takes four weeks, provided you have detoxed from chemicals first, during which you will be able to follow your normal working schedule, although having some extra time for leisurely baths, massage, skin brushing and other aids would certainly be a helpful bonus.

IS FASTING NECESSARY?

Fasting is a universal and ancient way to achieve natural healing. Animals instinctively stop eating when they are ill, and most, if not all, religious faiths have a tradition of fasting at certain times. Strictly speaking, fasting means eating and drinking nothing but water while the fast lasts. Recently, fasting has been used less frequently, partly because we tend to be overloaded with toxins and the withdrawal symptoms can be severe.

Some doctors consider that fasting is unwise; they believe that a minimum intake of protein is required for the liver to repair itself, as very little protein is stored in our bodies. Other doctors and naturopaths prescribe modified fasts that permit fruit juices. Dr William Rea, who specializes in treating patients with severe allergies and chemical sensitivities, prescribes fasting as therapy for many of his patients. He believes that there are benefits to be gained from skipping even one or two meals. You will find some information about mini-fasts in this book, but they are not an essential part of a detoxification programme.

WHAT HAPPENS IF YOU ARE ALREADY THIN AND DO NOT WANT TO LOSE WEIGHT?

Thin people often have the sort of metabolism that means that they can eat plenty of calories without gaining weight; conversely, they may lose weight too rapidly when they eat less.

People who are thin have to be careful NOT to lose weight while detoxing, and it is important for them to eat enough to make up for the calories that

WILL I LOSE WEIGHT?

A detoxification programme is not a weight loss programme. Indeed, some of the people who most benefit from detox are thin. However, if you do need to lose weight, you will almost certainly find that you shed a few pounds while detoxing, much of which is surplus water. In addition, the detox programmes restrict the intake of fatty and high-calorie foods. You will find several weight loss tips and ideas in Part Two of this book.

Many people find that once they have followed a detox programme it is relatively easy to continue with a weight loss programme as food cravings are less marked. In addition, you will have started to exercise on a regular basis, and there is no doubt that exercise enhances a reduced-calorie diet. It is not so much because you burn off the calories, but because exercise increases the rate that your body burns up energy, and this effect can last for several hours after exercise.

they usually obtain from sugar and alcohol. Very thin people find that, after detoxing, it is easier to maintain the weight that they desire, as their bodies tend to adjust to the correct weight for their body type.

IS COLONIC IRRIGATION NECESSARY?

The use of enemas and colonic irrigation for detoxing is controversial, although naturopaths have used both methods for internal cleansing for many years. In recent years, fibre supplements taken by mouth have been used to achieve the same purpose, mainly because irrigation has some risks and should certainly not be undertaken unless it is advised by a skilled, qualified therapist.

PART TWO

How to detox

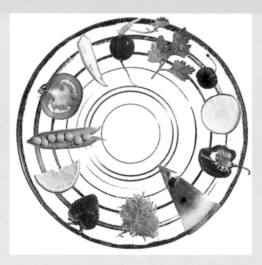

Following a detox programme is like emerging from a cold, dark winter's day into the spring sunshine.

Your **detox programmes**

Once you have decided to detox, choose the programme that will suit you best. Even a month is a relatively short investment in time to restore energy and a better level of health, and to give you a new start in life.

Within the 30-Day Makeover programme you will find a number of alternative choices so that you can vary the intensity of the programme to meet your needs, but even the most rigorous of these is compatible with a normal work routine. One advantage of several weeks spent detoxing is that you will find that your palate adapts to healthier food and you will be less likely to return to an unhealthy diet.

If you are in a hurry you could consider Detox in Nine Days, but this is a tougher programme. You will need a free week in which to take things easy, and you will probably develop marked side effects or withdrawal symptoms unless you already have a healthy lifestyle or have detoxed before. To maximize the benefit of this programme, it is best to make a commitment to continue with a lo-tox lifestyle and on-going maintenance programme (see Part Three).

If you are very busy and can devote only a few days at a time, the Weekend Energizer may be the perfect programme for you. With minimum input on Friday and a gentle dietary restriction on Monday, you can pack a lot of detoxing into a short time. Some people treat themselves to a Weekend Energizer every time the season changes.

If you are the type of person who thrives on a 'little and often' approach to staying healthy, or if you have only the occasional day for detoxing, have a look at the mini-fast and mono-diet programmes. You only have to commit yourself for a day, or even less, at any one time. Despite being so short, these programmes can make a real difference to the way you feel if they are repeated regularly.

CHEMICAL DETOXING

Unless you already have an extremely healthy lifestyle, it is likely that you consume some caffeine or sugar on a fairly regular basis. You may feel that you could easily do without these, but have you tried?

CHOOSING A PROGRAMME

- The 30-Day Makeover is a gentle first-time detox programme.

- The Weekend Energizer is ideal for busy people who have hectic schedules.

- Detox in Nine Days is a strict and intensive regime for those who wish to detox rapidly.

- Mini-fasts and mono-diets are effective short-term programmes that last one or two days.

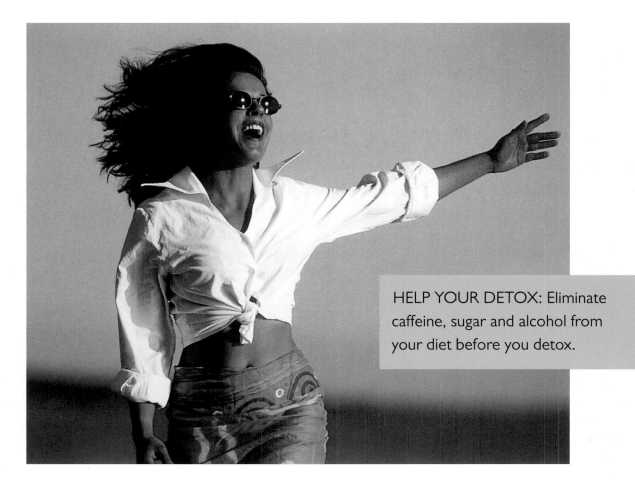

HELP YOUR DETOX: Eliminate caffeine, sugar and alcohol from your diet before you detox.

Many people have unpleasant withdrawal symptoms when they suddenly stop taking these substances and it is recommended that you withdraw from them gradually before starting a detox programme. Other chemicals can also cause problems, and you will find detoxing easier if, in advance of your detox programme, you also stop taking alcohol, recreational and over-the-counter drugs and tobacco.

CONSULTING YOUR DOCTOR

If you are generally feeling unwell or have any definite symptoms, you should consult your doctor before detox so that any underlying illness can be excluded. If you are pregnant, are regularly taking any prescribed medicine or have any medical condition, it is essential to obtain your doctor's agreement before undertaking your chosen detox programme. Many common conditions such as high blood pressure, raised cholesterol levels, allergies and diabetes can be improved by detoxing, but it is important to work with your doctor, who may need to change dosages of medication or provide you with extra guidance so that you can detox safely.

SIDE EFFECTS AND WITHDRAWAL SYMPTOMS

Almost everyone experiences some side effects during a detox. One cause is a sudden change in diet. You are likely to be eating less and your body will need a few

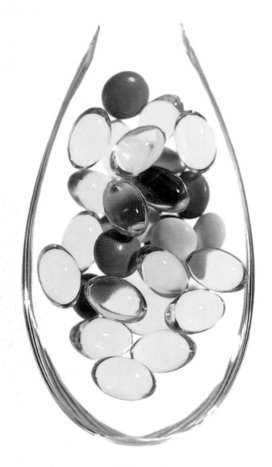

The side effects and withdrawal symptoms usually peak after about 48 hours, and go completely after five or six days, when most people report feeling much better and more energetic. The shorter detox programmes do not last this long, but if they are repeated on a regular basis, the feelings of well-being will occur more gradually, generally without you having to put up with the more intense symptoms. Repeating these programmes can be just as effective as a longer detox and provides a way to alter and enhance your lifestyle without making major changes all at once.

DETOX SUPPORTS

In addition to reducing the amount of chemicals you are putting into your body, your detox programme provides your body with high-quality nutrients to enhance the process. You can also choose to add extra vitamins and minerals (pp. 122–123), and herbal supplements that enhance liver function (pp. 74–76).

You can also take certain measures to help your body to dispose of toxins, such as brushing your skin, taking regular exercise and avoiding constipation. Before you start your detox programme, read through some of the suggestions in this chapter to decide which supports may be of most help to you. To improve your ability to cope with stress, you can 'detox your mind' with relaxation exercises and meditation (pp. 102–103). Finally, you can reduce the total load of chemicals that your body has to deal with by detoxing your environment (pp. 104–109). This does not mean that you have to make a great effort or spend a lot of money. There are many small ways to reduce environmental pollution that are easy and free and may even save you money.

days to adapt. In addition, however, you will be taking in fewer toxic chemicals, and you may develop symptoms as your body uses the opportunity to mobilize and detox chemicals that it has previously tucked away out of harm's way, usually in the fatty tissue of the body.

Many people are 'addicted' to certain foods. These foods are often the ones that they eat most frequently and may be the result of unrecognized food intolerance (see p. 88). When these foods are not supplied, the absence of some of the 'comfort' chemicals that these foods produce in our brains may cause cravings to develop. When you start to detox, your body needs a few days to adapt to these changes, too.

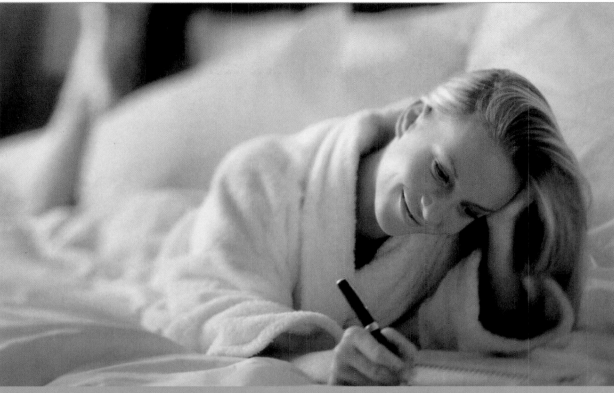

FOOD, MOOD AND EXERCISE **DIARIES**

Some people find that keeping a food, mood and exercise diary is very useful because it teaches them about themselves and helps them to understand the triggers that lead them to make unhealthy choices. There is growing scientific evidence that people who are trying to lose weight or break unhealthy habits, such as smoking, are more likely to succeed if they keep a diary. Even though they are only admitting their failures and successes to an entirely private document, it can still provide sufficient impetus for people to make healthy choices in their lifestyles.

Your diary does not have to be elaborate. A notebook that is large enough for you to draw three columns should be adequate. The left-hand column will be used for making a note of the time, but the other two should be wide enough to jot down a few lines.

In the middle column, write down what you eat, how much exercise you take or when you smoke; and in the right-hand column make brief notes about your mood at the time and any noticeable changes that occur. If you keep such a diary conscientiously, it will help you to analyse:

- When and where you are most likely to crave certain foods, a cigarette, an alcoholic drink or indulge whatever your weakness is. You can take steps to avoid any triggers.
- How you feel before and after; this may help if you think you are intolerant to certain foods (see p. 88), and to help you become aware of what enhances or depresses your moods.
- The times that exercise seems to help you most or your reasons for failing to do it.

Addictions: **chemical detox**

We become addicted to various chemicals because they can alter our mood and energy levels in the short term, but they add to the workload of our detox systems and eventually make us feel tired and stressed.

WATER OF LIFE: Drink plenty of water each day to make a major contribution to the success of your detox programme.

KICKING THE CAFFEINE HABIT

Caffeine can cross the placenta to an unborn baby during pregnancy and it is also secreted in breast milk. It is, therefore, often the first stimulant of childhood, and older children continue to obtain caffeine from cola drinks and chocolate. Many adults drink coffee, tea or chocolate drinks each day, often accompanied by sugar (see p. 36), and nicotine (see p. 42). Too much caffeine in our system can lead to fatigue, and the addictive cycle starts if more caffeine is then taken as a further stimulus. As our body adapts to caffeine (see below), greater amounts are needed to produce the same degree of stimulation, and the daily dose often increases every time we feel stressed or have problems to deal with.

CAFFEINE: THE DOWN SIDE

Caffeine raises blood pressure, increases heart rate and the levels of cholesterol in the blood. It can lead to sugar cravings and digestive upsets, including diarrhoea. If taken at or near meal times, caffeine can interfere with the absorption of calcium and iron, increasing the risks of osteoporosis and anaemia. Caffeine increases the production of urine, which may result in the loss of various minerals and vitamins. Symptoms from caffeine include anxiety, panic attacks, insomnia and, in children, hyperactivity.

In some women, caffeine appears to cause breast cysts, and pregnant mothers who take caffeine may have babies with low birth weights. In the United States, the Food and Drug Administration advises minimal intake of caffeine in pregnancy, because caffeine can cause birth deformities in animals, although this has not been shown in humans. It is thought that excess caffeine may increase the risk of certain cancers and the formation of kidney stones.

DETOX SLOWLY

Abrupt withdrawal from caffeine can cause headaches, fatigue, depression, poor concentration, digestive disturbance and changes in sleep. It is best to reduce your intake slowly over a couple of weeks.

LO-TOX MAINTENANCE (see also Part Three)

Once you have weaned yourself off caffeine and completed your detox programme, you will be used to living without this stimulus. However, you may feel that complete abstinence is hampering your social life or depriving you of pleasure. Up to about 100mg per day is unlikely to cause ill effects, but to make sure that you are not becoming addicted again, have a caffeine-free week every two to three months. If this causes recurrence of withdrawal symptoms, you should reduce your intake of caffeine permanently.

DETOX SUPPORTS

Common sources of caffeine	Typical dose per 180ml/6oz
Fresh coffee	80–150mg
Instant coffee	60–70mg
Decaffeinated coffee*	up to 10mg
Tea	45–55mg
Cocoa or hot chocolate	20–30mg
Cola drinks	30–50mg
Certain medicines such as pain killers and cold remedies	(up to 200mg per dose; check label)

* Check the process used for removing caffeine. Steaming is safe, but other methods may leave behind chemical residues.

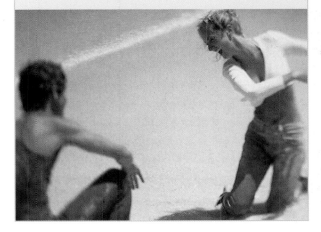

LIVING WITHOUT REFINED SUGAR

For many people, especially those with a sweet tooth, the abrupt removal of refined sugar from their diet during a dietary detox programme can cause unpleasant symptoms. These occur because our bodies were not designed to deal with the large amount of refined sugar that is often present in Western diets today. Eating too much sugar is thought to contribute to the development of diabetes in older age and hypoglycaemia (low level of sugar in the blood). In both these conditions, the body's normally tight control of the level of sugar in the blood is lost to a greater or lesser extent.

Nutritional scientists recommend eating a maximum of about 60g/2oz per day of the types of sugar that have been defined as 'extrinsic', excluding those in milk. These are sugars that are not contained within the cell walls of the food that is being eaten. Fruit juice, therefore, has to be counted as part of the maximum intake, whereas whole fruit does not. This allowance may sound generous, but if you read food labels you will see that many foods, even savoury foods and meal substitutes designed for slimmers, contain 30g/1oz per portion.

LOW BLOOD SUGAR (HYPOGLYCAEMIA)

Refined sugars are generally absorbed quickly from the intestine, and the pancreas responds by secreting large amounts of insulin. This pushes sugar into the body's cells, reducing the level in the blood, where it can cause damage. But about three to five hours after a meal the blood sugar level may be low enough to cause symptoms such as migraines, feelings of weakness, light-headedness, confusion or aggression.

Fortunately, hypoglycaemia can be overcome by eating more whole grains, brown rice and pasta, with a limited amount of whole fruit, and by following an exercise programme (see pp. 90–91). Whole foods reduce sugar craving by supplying chromium, which helps to regulate insulin secretion. Eating a piece of whole fruit, excluding bananas, 30–60 minutes before a meal can reduce sugar cravings and, in slimmers, help to reduce appetite.

SUGAR CRAVINGS

There is a growing body of scientific evidence supporting the theory that you can become truly addicted to sugar. Sugar releases some of the naturally occurring chemicals in our brain that calm mood and decrease sensitivity to pain, both physical and emotional. Some of us appear to have an inborn deficit of these chemicals, and as a result we crave sugar because it makes us feel better.

If you are a sugar-craver, you should certainly cut down on your sugar intake before embarking on a dietary detox programme to minimize withdrawal symptoms, and you may find it best to have a separate 'sugar detox', too.

THE SUGAR DETOX

If you eat a lot of sugar, cut down gradually over a few weeks and then completely stop eating it. If you have a sweet tooth, but your sugar intake has been largely controlled by willpower and/or you are in a hurry, just stop eating sugar. For the first five or six days you are likely to experience symptoms such as nausea, diarrhoea, irritability and headaches. So choose a time when these will not disrupt an important

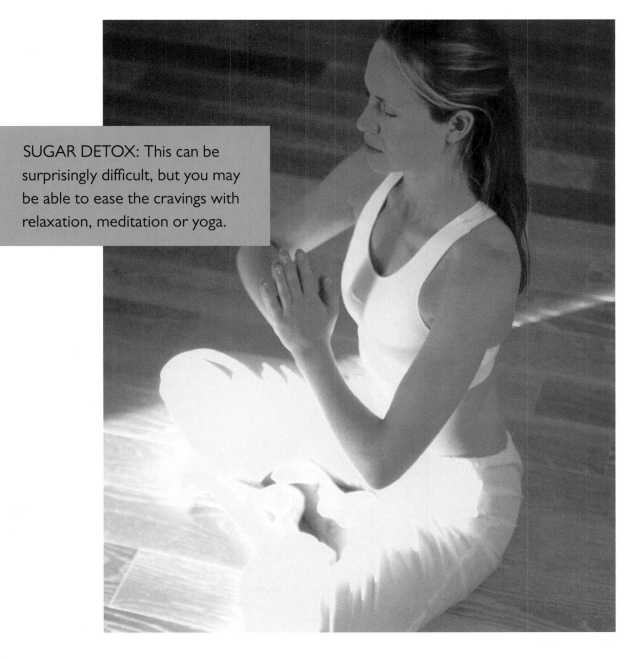

SUGAR DETOX: This can be surprisingly difficult, but you may be able to ease the cravings with relaxation, meditation or yoga.

engagement or celebration. You can help to reduce the severity of your symptoms by drinking plenty of water, six to eight glasses each day. You should avoid replacing sugar with fat or alcohol. Don't drink fruit juice during the sugar detox, and limit yourself to two pieces of whole fruit a day if you become desperate, but it is probably better not to eat any at all until you are through the worst symptoms. Avoid artificial sweeteners, as they will only perpetuate your longing for sweet things.

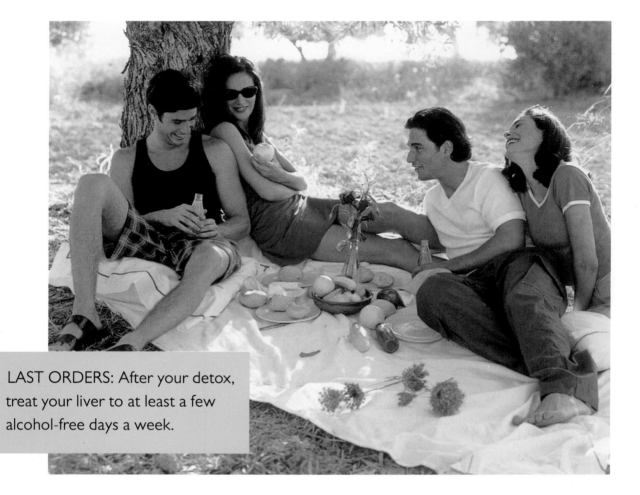

LAST ORDERS: After your detox, treat your liver to at least a few alcohol-free days a week.

THE TROUBLE WITH ALCOHOL

Alcohol, even in moderate amounts, can cause a number of problems. Not only does alcohol interfere with the absorption of some important nutrients, but the liver also needs an extra supply of nutrients to break down alcohol into its safer components of carbon dioxide and water. Indeed, doing this is so vital that the liver detoxifies alcohol as a priority and may put off other important functions when alcohol is present.

Although most people can handle one or two drinks a day safely, having a few alcohol-free days each week allows your body to recover, and reduces the risks to health from alcohol. These include liver disease, heart disease, inflammation and ulceration of the stomach, hypoglycaemia and diabetes, inflammation of the pancreas, disorders of the nervous system, obesity, suppression of the immune system, impotence and birth defects. Saving up your two daily drinks and having them all at the weekend can undo the good you have done yourself by abstaining, because your liver will be overwhelmed. Not only will you have alcohol and its poisonous breakdown products circulating around your body, but your liver will also be unable to perform its normal functions.

ALCOHOL AND DIETARY DETOXING

Complete abstinence is, of course, a part of any dietary detox. If you feel you couldn't survive for a few days without drinking alcohol, you may have an alcohol problem and should seek professional advice. Medical advice is essential before attempting dietary detox if:

- You have been drinking a bottle of wine, half a bottle of spirits or a six-pack of beer every day for a year or so, or
- You have ever had problems, such as fits, the DTs, depression or agitation, when stopping alcohol, or
- You take any drugs as well as more than two alcoholic drinks a day.

If you have been regularly drinking more than three drinks a day you should plan to cut down before beginning your dietary detox. During this time, your liver will benefit if you eat a nutritious diet (see Part Three) and take a good multi-mineral and vitamin supplement.

LO-TOX MAINTENANCE

Many people find the idea of complete abstinence from alcohol, except during a dietary detox, unacceptable as it would disrupt their social lives, and it can be argued that alcohol does have some benefits. Drinking a couple of glasses of wine with a meal can help with digestion and, since the meal delays the absorption of the alcohol, the liver has time to deal with it gradually.

Red wine also provides proanthocyanidins (OPCs) which act with vitamin C to remove the dangerous chemicals, known as free radicals, before they can cause any harm.

AVOIDING 'EMPTY CALORIES'

'Empty calories' come from foods that are sources of energy, but that contain no other nutrients, such as minerals and vitamins. The best example is white sugar, which has been refined from sugar cane or beet. The nutrient-rich molasses that has been left behind after the sugar has been removed can be used as a sweetener when its stronger taste is not a problem, such as in gingerbread or other spicy food.

Calories from alcohol are not entirely 'empty'. In addition to OPCs (which you can obtain from grapes or their juice), some wines contain vitamin C and beers contain B-vitamins. However, the amount of these nutrients is tiny when compared to the number of calories that alcohol provides (almost double the calories from carbohydrate or protein).

Worse still, calories that are derived from alcohol tend to be transformed into fat that is stored as fatty tissue and in the liver, unless your overall calorie intake is low. If this is the case, you are likely to be eating a diet that is deficient in other nutrients.

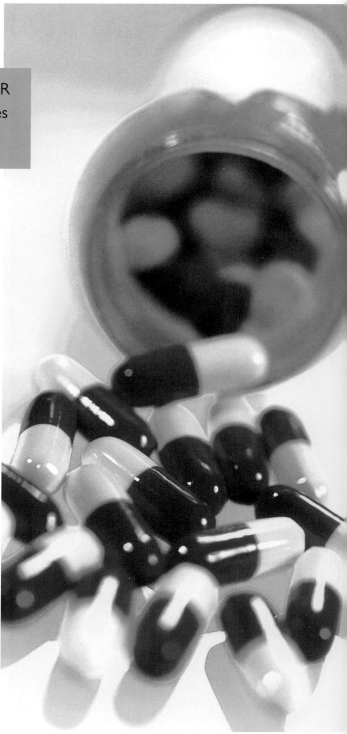

AVOID OVER-THE-COUNTER MEDICATION: Use alternatives where possible.

THE DRUG DETOX

All drugs put a strain on the liver. Many drugs lead to addiction, which means that increased doses are needed to maintain the same effect, and withdrawal symptoms occur when we try to give them up. If your liver is overworked and under stress, it may not detoxify drugs fully and breakdown products can accumulate in fatty tissue. Sometimes the breakdown products are themselves toxic, and they can cause symptoms and even poison the liver, causing it to function less efficiently.

OVER-THE-COUNTER MEDICINES

Abuse of over-the-counter medicines often goes unrecognized because they can be obtained legally and are generally less toxic than other drugs. They are often taken for the relief of acute symptoms such as headaches, or allergic symptoms such as sneezing or a runny nose. Unfortunately, painkillers can sometimes be the cause of the regular headaches they are taken to alleviate, and it is easy to end up taking them daily or several times a week. In general, you should try to find natural therapies such as nutritional supplements, herbs, homeopathy or naturopathy to improve your health, and avoid chemical medicines as much as possible, as these increase the work of the detox systems (see above).

PRESCRIBED MEDICINES

Some doctors tend to overestimate the usefulness of conventional medicines, but conversely, alternative practitioners may underestimate their value. It is important to seek advice from the practitioner who prescribed your medicine before you stop taking it or alter the dose in any way. If you are taking prescribed medication or have any medical condition, you should discuss your detox programme with your doctor. You may also need to consult your doctor again as your detox programme progresses, because the doses of your medication may need to be adjusted. For example, your blood pressure or the level of cholesterol in your blood may drop low enough for you to reduce or even discontinue your medication.

STREET AND RECREATIONAL DRUGS

The first steps towards withdrawing from the regular use of hard drugs and tranquillizers requires a recognition that these substances can cause serious harm, and the courage to ask for help from your doctor. Some of these drugs cannot be stopped immediately without risk. Any detox programme should be professionally supervised so that withdrawal is gradual and other supportive medication and herbal preparations can be used. Unless you are advised otherwise, you can help to reduce the withdrawal symptoms by eating a diet rich in fruit and vegetables.

GETTING OFF **DRUGS**

Ask for your doctor's advice about withdrawing from over-the-counter and recreational drugs and stop them before starting the detox programme that you have chosen. A number of drugs, especially marijuana, are stored in the body fat and withdrawal can lead to flashbacks and other ongoing symptoms, so give yourself time. You can accelerate the process of withdrawal by sweating, either from exercise, saunas or other appropriate hydrotherapy measures (see pp. 94–97), by losing weight, or by taking herbs such as goldenseal, dandelion or milk thistle (see pp. 74–76). If you feel agitated, valerian may help (p. 76), but do not drive or operate machinery. If you are uncertain about the best dose of any herbal preparation, seek professional advice.

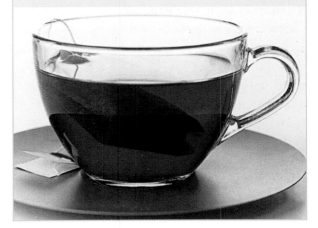

GIVING UP TOBACCO

Tobacco smoke contains more than 4,000 chemicals, of which over 50 are known to cause cancer. In addition, smoking is a major cause of heart disease. You will already know this, yet you continue to smoke. This is because smoking is addictive. Like sugar, smoking can enhance the production of the naturally occurring chemicals in the brain that calm mood and decrease sensitivity to pain, both physical and emotional. Ideally, you should give up smoking before a dietary detox, but if you find this impossible cut down as much as you can.

PLAN YOUR SMOKING DETOX

Many doctors believe that the single most effective detox measure that smokers can undertake is to give up smoking. Few people find it easy, but there are ways and means of doing it. You may decide which day you will give up, and then just do it. You know that the withdrawal symptoms won't last forever, and that you will soon feel better.

Alternatively, you can choose a two-stage operation. First, stop smoking and then withdraw from nicotine, using either nicotine patches or gum. If you note down the times you want a cigarette in your food, mood and exercise diary (see p. 33) you will be able to work out whether there are definite triggers to your smoking, such as driving the car or following a meal, in which case replacing the cigarette with gum can help beat the cravings. If your smoking pattern is more haphazard, you may prefer to use a patch which provides a steady release of nicotine.

After a while, you become accustomed to not smoking, find other ways to relax, avoid places where

PASSIVE **SMOKING**

Even if you don't smoke, your health can be damaged by the passive inhalation of tobacco smoke. Non-smokers are more sensitive to smoke than regular smokers are, and environmental smoke has been shown to have a higher concentration of some toxic chemicals.

Passive smokers can protect themselves to some extent by taking antioxidant nutrients such as vitamins C and E.

Smokers can also be motivated to give up to prevent a child or a loved one from suffering the ill effects of passive smoking. There is now some evidence to support the belief that parents can protect their unborn children if they both give up smoking at least three months before a planned conception. The cell divisions needed to produce sperm take three months to be completed, and the father may damage this delicate process if he smokes.

The same three months allows the mother's body to detox from cigarette smoke and to make good any nutritional deficiency that has resulted from smoking.

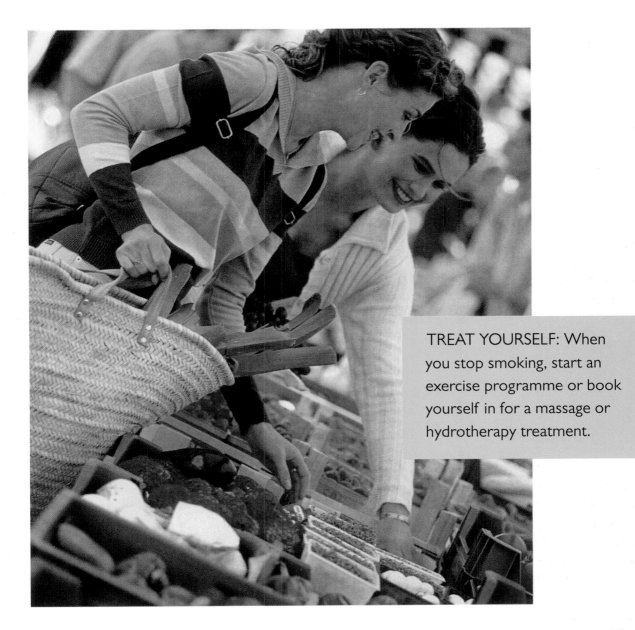

TREAT YOURSELF: When you stop smoking, start an exercise programme or book yourself in for a massage or hydrotherapy treatment.

you might be tempted to smoke and take one day at a time. If you wish, join a support group. Once you are through the worst, start reducing your dose of nicotine: do not leave this for too long as the nicotine is still giving your liver extra work. Motivate yourself with rewards by spending the money you have saved on something that you really want, but try to avoid food rewards, as you do not want to put on weight.

When you stop smoking, eat as healthily as you can (see Part Three) to make up nutritional deficiencies and allow your body to repair any damage that smoking has caused. Take a good mineral and vitamin supplement, start an exercise programme (pp. 90–91) and use some of the hydrotherapy suggestions (pp. 94–97).

The dietary **detox programmes**

The 30-Day Makeover Programme

This programme is designed as a gentle first-time detox, but it contains options that are more rigorous if you have been doing one or more of the shorter programmes or if you already have a very healthy lifestyle.

You can continue to go to work, but if possible choose a month that is not too busy so that you can devote time to relaxation, exercise and massage. The programme has been arranged so that you can start on a Saturday. You may find it helpful to tell your work colleagues what you are doing and ask for their support. If you have unavoidable social engagements, try to enlist the support of your host or hostess so that you can continue your detox. But if all else fails you can follow the Emergency Plan (see box, p. 46), which will extend the programme by two days each time you have to use it.

WHAT YOU CAN EAT AND DRINK
You should not be hungry (except at the weekends if you choose the more rigorous, Optional Intensive Plan, p. 48). You can eat three meals and up to three snacks each day: although your choice of food is limited, the amount you can eat is not. Slimmers, however, should limit the amount of olive oil used in dressings.

The diet for the 30-Day Makeover programme is based on generous portions of vegetables and fruit, with some protein and modest amounts of fat. Eat vegetables and fruit raw or lightly cooked so that it is as fresh as possible and, preferably, organically grown. In particular, eat two or more servings every day that are rich in carotenoids and vitamin C.

Carotenoids are found in orange, red and green fruit and vegetables such as carrots, sweet potatoes, spinach, melons, apricots, peaches, winter squash, tomato purée, spring greens, watercress, broccoli and Brussels sprouts. Carotenoids can be destroyed by heat processes such as canning, boiling or steaming; and also by air and light, as when fruits are dried in the sun. Always try to eat these foods fresh, and raw or cooked lightly.

Vitamin C is contained in citrus fruits, kiwi fruit, blackcurrants, broccoli, tomato purée, strawberries, raw cabbage, bell peppers, parsley and guavas. Vitamin C is lost from food when it is cooked at high temperatures and during storage, so, again, try to eat these foods fresh, either cooked briefly or raw.

WHAT TO AVOID
The 30-Day Makeover programme excludes the foods that most commonly cause food intolerance (see pp. 88–89), such as wheat, cows' milk and milk products,

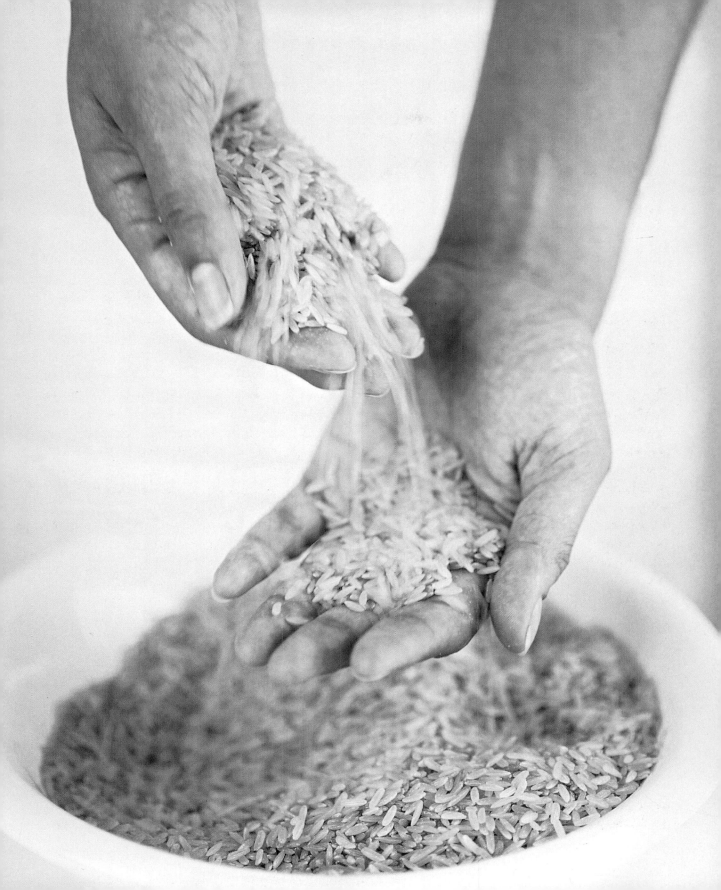

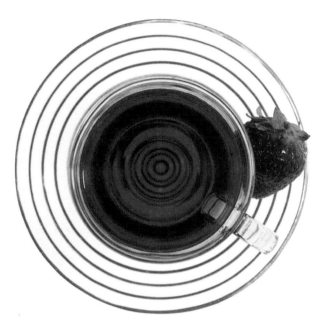

EMERGENCY **PLAN**

BEFORE GOING TO BED

• Drink at least 600ml/1 pint of water (flavoured with juice from a lime or lemon if preferred), or dandelion tea.

• Take a strong B-complex supplement and 1000mg of vitamin C.

DURING THE NEXT TWO DAYS

• Take extra vitamin C and follow week one of the Makeover programme for two days. Then return to where you were on the programme.

previously excluded foods, you should avoid them throughout the programme (see Intolerance, pp. 88–89, and Maintenance in Part Three).

PREPARING FOR YOUR MAKEOVER

In the week before you start the Makeover programme, read through the sections on detox supports, herbs and supplements (see pp. 74–76) and stock up on items that you will need, such as a skin brush, aromatherapy and massage oils, salts for hydrotherapy, and your chosen supplements. Try to borrow a juicer and food processor if you don't own them. Dietary basics include cold pressed olive oil, bottled still mineral water (or a new filter for your jug) and other drinks such as herbal teas (see p. 77), and dandelion tea and coffee (see p. 75). Try to eat a light diet for a few days before starting, and have an early night on the Friday.

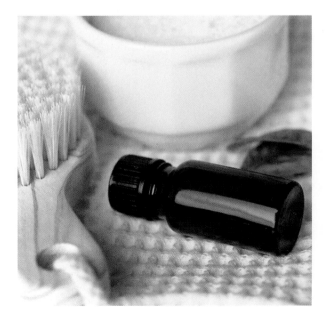

eggs, sugar and artificial sweeteners, as well as alcohol, caffeine and soft drinks. You should also avoid foods that are high in fat or salt, or contain artificial flavourings, colourings and preservatives. Do not eat any foods that you know you do not tolerate well. The first week is strict, but extra choices are introduced each week. If you develop any symptoms after eating

BASIC DAILY TIMETABLE FOR THE **MAKEOVER PROGRAMME**

On waking	Drink one to two glasses of warm water flavoured with fresh lime or lemon juice. Do some stretching exercises. Take a bath or shower, with skin brushing (see p. 94) if you have time.
Breakfast	Have breakfast from foods allowed.
Mid-morning drink	Lime or lemon water, vegetable juice (see p. 69), or dandelion tea or coffee. You may have a piece of fruit or some crudités if you are hungry. You should not have any fruit juice for the first two weeks of your detox.
Pre-lunch drink	Have water or maybe a herbal tea that helps digestion, such as peppermint or fennel, about half an hour before lunch. If you prefer, boil slices of ginger in a cup of water, adjusting the amount to your taste, or make a herbal infusion (see p. 77). Both of these can be made in advance before you go to work and kept in a vacuum flask (either hot or chilled).
Lunch	Eat your lunch without drinking at the same time, as there is plenty of water in your fruit and vegetables and extra will dilute your digestive juices. Have a period of relaxation (see pp. 100–101). If you are at work, try to spend a few minutes quietly out of doors.
Mid-afternoon drink	Lime or lemon water, herb tea or vegetable juice. Have a piece of fruit or some crudités if you are hungry, or a rosemary infusion if you feel tired or have a headache (see p. 76).
Exercise	Build up slowly if you haven't been doing very much (see p. 90). Avoid heavy exercise during any weekend when you follow the optional programme. Have a drink half an hour before your evening meal, as at lunchtime.
Evening meal	Eat your evening meal as early as possible to allow digestion to be complete before you go to bed. Avoid drinking any fluid with it. Have a bath or hydrotherapy (see pp. 94–97). Try to go to bed early. You can drink a relaxing tea such as chamomile, or take a valerian supplement. If you are hungry, have a piece of fruit or some crudités.

Optional **Intensive Plan**

If you have detoxed before, or have not been experiencing more than five symptoms every day (see questionnaire, pp. 22–23), why not make an extra effort over one or more of the weekends of your makeover?

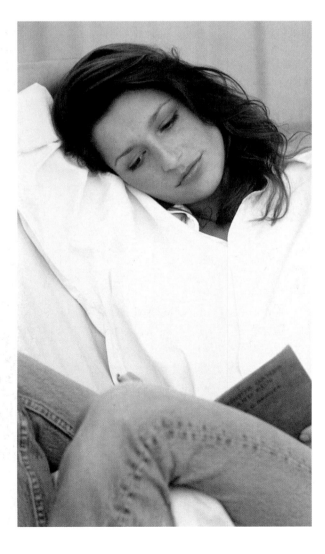

Some of you might prefer to 'kick start' your detox by following a more intensive programme; alternatively you could put aside a special weekend later in the detox programme: clear your diary and really pamper yourself by eating lightly and undertaking only gentle activity. If this is your first detox, you will probably find that following each week's diets is sufficiently challenging for the moment. You can always plan Weekend Energizers (see p. 64), mini-fasts (see pp. 70–72) or mono-diet days (see pp. 70–73) as part of your maintenance programme (see Part Three).

For your intensive weekend detox choose one of the following:

- One or two days of mono-diet (see pp. 70–72).
- Mini-fasting for one or both days (see pp. 70–73).
- Fasting on Saturday and eating fruit and vegetables that are raw or lightly cooked on Sunday.

Your one-day fast can be a water-only fast, you can add a little lemon or lime for flavour if you wish, or you can drink potassium broth (see box) or vegetable juices. Drink some liquid every two hours, or more frequently if you are thirsty. You should drink at least ten glasses of fluid, but not more than 20. Try to sip and move your drinks around your mouth to keep it fresh. On the second day eat raw fruit and vegetables.

POTASSIUM **BROTH**

- Chop up about 1.5kg/3lb of mixed vegetables, organic if possible. They should be well washed and the root vegetables scrubbed: do not peel them if they are organic.

- Add a bunch of parsley and include beetroot and turnip tops if you have them.

- Place them in a stainless steel or pyrex saucepan with 2.2¼pt of filtered or spring water, but do not add seasoning.

- Bring to the boil and simmer gently for 30 minutes.

- Leave to cool and then strain off the liquid and store it in the fridge until you need it.

If you find them difficult to digest they can be lightly cooked. As throughout the Makeover programme you should include fruit and vegetables that are rich in carotenoids and vitamin C (see p. 44).

FOR YOUR SAFETY AND COMFORT

During a fast or mono-diet, it is important to rest and to wear warm clothes if you feel cold. Do NOT drive or operate machinery while fasting. The first time you fast, you are likely to feel a little muzzy and have a furred tongue. Your sweat may smell unpleasant and you may wish to shower or bath more frequently than usual, but avoid having hot bath. (See also side effects and withdrawal symptoms, pp. 82–85.) Gentle exercise can be taken, preferably in the fresh air.

The presence of withdrawal symptoms or side effects is a sign that the detox is working, and each time you fast or restrict your diet these symptoms are likely to be less severe. For this reason, it is often a good idea to start with the gentlest approach and increase the intensity of your weekend programmes as your health improves. If you are going to work on the Monday, be sure to include plenty of starchy vegetables in your evening meal on Sunday.

Week **one**

During the first week your diet is restricted and simple. The aim is to give your body a real rest from having to digest and process foods that have low nutritional value, such as refined sugar and alcohol, or none at all, such as food additives.

SHOPPING LIST FOR WEEK I

- Brown rice, quinoa, millet, buckwheat, including their flours, flakes and egg-free pastas.
- Rice cakes and crackers, puffed rice cereal.
- Fresh fruit (at least two to four servings daily) and vegetables (at least three to five servings daily): choose your favourites, but be sure to include a wide variety (see super vegetables, p. 78), and some of those listed on p. 44, which contain carotenoids and vitamin C. This week you should cut out members of the potato family (potatoes, tomatoes, peppers, aubergines): sweet potatoes, peas and root vegetables make filling alternatives.
- Herbs, fresh if possible, and spices for flavouring.
- Avoid salt if you can.
- Fish, fresh or frozen, but if this is not possible have tinned fish in water or brine, but not in oil. Avoid smoked fish.
- Rice milk. If you cannot buy it without additives, make your own by adding one mug of cooked rice to four mugs of mineral or filtered water, plus a teaspoonful of vanilla essence if desired. Blend or liquidize until smooth, stand for an hour, and then strain through a sieve. Chill in the fridge, then shake well before using.
- Lemons or limes to flavour your water.
- Olive oil.

DIETARY GUIDE FOR WEEK I

It is important to eat enough protein to repair your liver and immune system, so have fish once or twice every day. If you are a vegetarian or really dislike fish, eat plenty of the grains: both quinoa and millet contain complete protein (see p. 55 for cooking times). If you are concerned about your calcium intake without milk in your diet, check the list on p. 123 for other sources of calcium. Dress your salads with a little olive oil to which you can add lemon/lime juice and plenty of your favourite herbs.

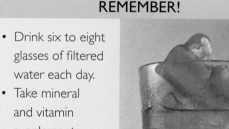

REMEMBER!

- Drink six to eight glasses of filtered water each day.
- Take mineral and vitamin supplements (pp. 122–123) and other herbal preparations (pp. 74–76) with meals.

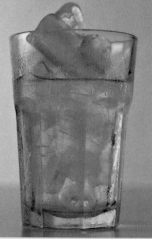

BREAKFAST SUGGESTIONS

Two pieces of fruit

Fruit smoothie: in a liquidizer, whizz together 250ml/8fl oz (one cup) rice milk, one banana and some berries or other fruit such as a stoned peach, or a cored pear.

Puffed rice and rice milk.

Porridge made from any allowed grains (see grain cooking times, p. 55).

Rice cakes and mashed banana.

LUNCH AND EVENING MEAL

Have one meal with a single course and one meal with two courses: if possible eat your two-course meal in the middle of the day.

Main course suggestions:

Vegetable curry or casserole on brown rice (you can include fish if you wish).

Rice or buckwheat pasta with baked fish and steamed vegetables or salad.

Grilled fish with a large helping of steamed vegetables and/or salad with an olive oil and lemon/lime juice vinaigrette.

Vegetable pilaf, including fish if desired; ring the changes by using millet or quinoa instead of rice (for cooking times, see p. 55).

Fish baked on a selection of pre-cooked vegetables.

- The second course can be eaten before or after the main course: ideally this should be vegetable based, for example, a large mixed salad or home-made vegetable soup, especially if you are snacking on fruit. If you crave something sweet, have half a grapefruit or chopped fruits served in their own juice.

MIND AND BODY **PLAN**

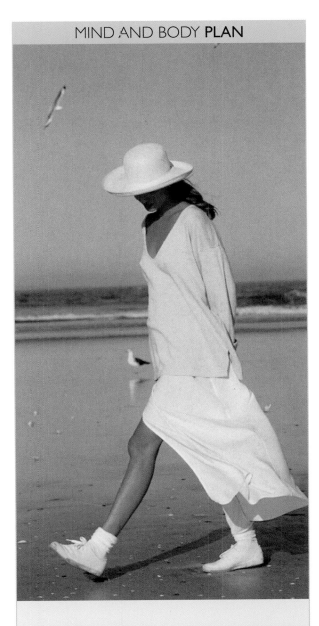

Walk for around 15 minutes each day in the fresh air. Enjoy leisurely baths with relaxing essential oils (p. 97). Start skin brushing (p. 94). Your diet is quite strict this week so exercise gently.

Week **two**

This week you can start to introduce some of the foods that were excluded last week. You should no longer be experiencing withdrawal symptoms or side effects and should be starting to feel the benefits of your detox.

Go on eating plenty of fresh produce each day: your goal is two to four pieces of fruit and three to five servings of vegetables.

Remember to drink lots of water every day and to take your supplements. If you want to lose weight you should stay on the week 2 diet plan for several weeks. It is a very healthy diet that is low in fat and contains generous amounts of fresh fruit and vegetables.

SHOPPING LIST FOR WEEK 2

In addition to your week 1 list you can now eat:

- Produce from the potato family: potatoes, tomatoes, peppers and aubergines, provided they do not cause allergy or intolerance (see pp. 88–89).
- Poultry: choose organic if possible and remove the skin before cooking, as it is high in saturated fat (see p. 121).
- Soy milk and soy products such as tofu and yoghurt.
- Seed and bean sprouts (see p. 63).
- Beans and lentils: these are filling foods that are rich in minerals as well as containing good-quality protein. If they give you wind (gas) try sprouting them before you cook them (see p. 55). If you are cooking dried beans soak them overnight and remember that all beans should be boiled briskly for ten minutes in an uncovered pan at the start of

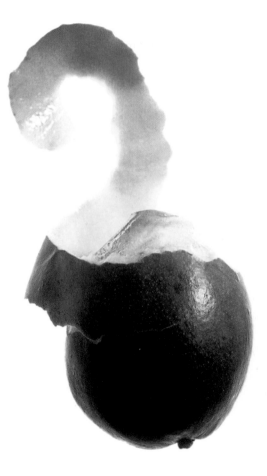

cooking. Beans freeze well, so you can save time by cooking them in bulk and freezing portions for use at a later date.

MENU SUGGESTIONS

For breakfast: you could experiment with eating fruits that perhaps you do not often have, such as papaya or mangoes. In your other meals, you can now include a baked potato once or twice in the week; use chicken in paella and risotto, but the only cheese you are allowed is dairy free, based on tofu. You can make your soups more filling by including lentils and beans.

THE SECOND WEEKEND.

Once again you may decide to follow the Optional Intensive Plan (pp. 48–49), before allowing yourself the greater food choices of week 2. Alternatively, give your detox a boost by having a glass of vegetable juice (see p. 64) instead of breakfast and your mid-morning and mid-afternoon drinks. This is a concentrated source of vegetable goodness, such as minerals, vitamins, bioflavonoids, and carotenoids (see p. 44) all of which deliver a real wake-up call to your liver and help it to function effectively.

DIETARY GUIDE FOR WEEK 2

You have an increased choice of food this week, which will make following your normal diet easier, but it is important to stay off common grains such as wheat, rye oats and barley. Do not skip breakfast: your body hasn't had any food for some hours and needs nourishment, not only to give you energy but also to jump-start your detox system. Even if you do not feel at all hungry, have some fruit or a fruit smoothie (p. 51) to help prevent the temptation to snack on cakes or chocolate later in the morning.

MIND AND BODY **PLAN**

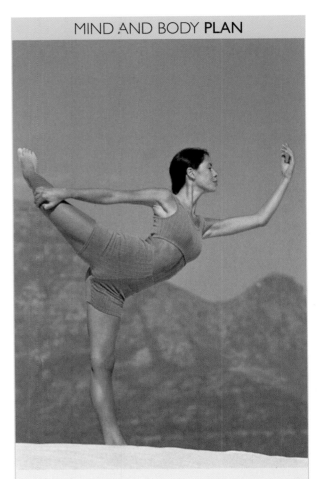

This week is the time to increase the amount of exercise you take so begin to be more adventurous with your stretching and yoga routines. Try to increase the amount of exercise that helps to promote healthy heart and lungs (see p. 91). It is a good time to book a relaxing massage or some aromatherapy. Read the suggestions for environmental detoxing (pp. 104–109) and consider how best to adopt some of the suggestions.

Week **three**

Congratulations! You are now halfway through The 30-Day Makeover Programme. Spend a few minutes this weekend with the questionnaire on pp. 22–23 to check out the improvement in your score.

THE THIRD WEEKEND

Once again, you can choose the Optional Intensive Plan (pp. 48–49), or drink freshly made vegetable juice as suggested for last weekend.

SHOPPING AND DIETARY GUIDE FOR WEEK 3

You can, of course, continue to eat the foods allowed during week 2, and this week you can also add:

- Nuts and nut milks: have these in moderation as they contain a high proportion of fat, even though it is mostly unsaturated (see p. 121).
- Sunflower, pumpkin and sesame seeds. These also contain unsaturated fat and can be sprouted before you eat them. Even if you do not have time to sprout them, try soaking sunflower and pumpkin seeds for 15–20 minutes before scattering them on a salad, as this makes them more crunchy.
- Fresh home-made fruit juices (if you have a yeast/candida problem, see p. 87). Fruit juice is a concentrated source of sugar and should be diluted with at least an equal volume of filtered or spring water. It is best to avoid commercial juices as they often have additives such as sugar, or contain yeasts which can be avoided when the juice is freshly prepared from fruit that is not over-ripe.
- Organically produced, free-range eggs.

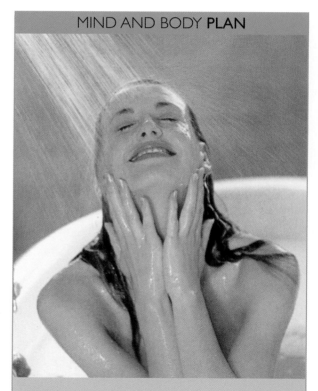

MIND AND BODY **PLAN**

Why not have one or two saunas this week? Alternatively, you can increase your detox through the skin by having an Epsom salt bath (see p. 96) or wet wrap (see p. 97). Continue to increase the amount of exercise you are taking, and make plans to continue this after the Makeover.

RECIPES

COOKING TIMES FOR GRAINS

Cooking times vary, as grains may be pre-treated in a number of ways, but some approximate times are given here if there are no instructions on the packet. The times can be reduced considerably if you pre-soak the grain.

Grain	Amount (Measures*)	Water (Measures*)	Cooking time (minutes)
Barley	1	3	20
Brown rice	1	2	35–40
Millet	1	3	35–40
Oats	1	2	45–60
Quinoa	1	2	15

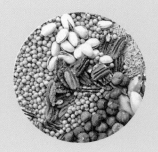

*A common measure is an American cup, but you can substitute a mug or teacup, or fill a measuring jug to the 250ml/8oz level, which is equivalent to an American cup. Adjust the number of measures you use to the number of people you are cooking for and the size of their appetites.

NUT AND SEED MILKS AND CREAMS

Proportions:

Nut cream	1 measure of nuts to 1 measure of water
Nut milk	1 measure of nuts to 2 measures of water
Sesame seed milk	1 measure of seeds to 4 measures of water
Sunflower seed milk	1 measure of seeds to 2 measures of water

NUT MILK AND CREAM

- Measure the water and either soak the nuts in it overnight, or bring it to the boil and blanch the nuts in it for two to three minutes.
- Drain the nuts, but the water.
- Place the nuts in a blender and grind coarsely.
- Add the water and blend with vanilla as desired.
- Store in the fridge if not using immediately.

SEED MILKS

Follow steps 3, 4 and 5. If it tastes a little bitter, you can add one or two stoned fresh dates.

Suitable nuts:

Almond, brazil, cashew.
Chestnut and water chestnut (good choices for slimmers as they contain less fat than most nuts. Dried chestnuts must be soaked overnight.)
Coconut (caution: high in saturated fat), hazel, macadamia, pecan, pinenut, pistachio and walnut.

Week **four**

Congratulations! You are now only one week away from completing The 30-Day Makeover Programme and you should be feeling more energetic and relaxed and experiencing fewer symptoms.

SHOPPING AND DIETARY GUIDE FOR WEEK 4

You can choose to follow the Optional Intensive Plan for the fourth weekend, or the vegetable juice booster suggested for the second weekend (see p. 53).

- Oats, barley, and rye can now be added to your diet. Oatcakes and crispbreads are good choices, but you should check the food labels as some varieties contain wheat or wheat bran. You should also continue to avoid rye bread that is made with sourdough, as this is a yeast.
- You can now have oatmeal porridge or sugar-free cornflakes for breakfast, and use barley in soups and casseroles.
- Treat yourself to lean, organic red meat if you enjoy meat, but avoid browning it in fat (see p. 120).
- Remember to eat oily fish once or twice a week, and even if you are not a vegetarian you should try to have one or two 'veggie' days each week (see protein, pp. 118–119).

THE FIFTH WEEKEND

You have now almost completed a 30-day detox programme. This weekend you can start to reintroduce cows' milk and milk products, and wheat, including products containing yeast, such as bread. If you think that you might be intolerant of any of these, you should introduce the wheat, yeast, and milk one at a time, with an interval of four days between each introduction (see pp. 88–89). For further suggestions on returning to your usual diet and adopting maintenance programmes that will extend the benefit from your detox, see Part Three.

This weekend is a good time to add up your score from the questionnaire on pp. 22–23 again. It should be markedly lower than when you started the programme, and you'll probably find you have shed a few pounds.

MIND AND BODY **PLAN**

By now, relaxation will be becoming easier as you have been practising it regularly. Try to continue taking a short relaxation period every day after the Makeover, as this will help you to cope with everyday stress and improve your efficiency at work. In addition, it can help with your physical health by reducing the risk of developing heart disease and digestive problems, and may also relieve insomnia.

IF YOU WANT TO **LOSE MORE WEIGHT**

If you want to lose more weight, this is an ideal time to follow a gentle weight-loss programme by continuing to eat a diet that is low in fat and high in fresh fruits and vegetables.

Aim to lose around 0.5–1kg/1–2lb a week. If you lose weight faster than this after the first couple of weeks of a diet (when the weight loss is mostly fluid), you are likely to lose muscle or lean tissue. This is not advisable because the basic rate at which your body burns up energy depends on the amount of muscle that you have. So if your body starts to break down muscle (to supply essential energy to your brain) you will find that losing weight and keeping it off becomes even more difficult.

To counteract this, continue taking regular exercise. The best regime for weight loss is long sessions, lasting 45–60 minutes, of not too intense exercise such as walking or cycling (see p. 91) three to five days a week, but not every day as your muscles and joints need to rest. Swimming seems less effective for weight loss, but it is good for a healthy heart.

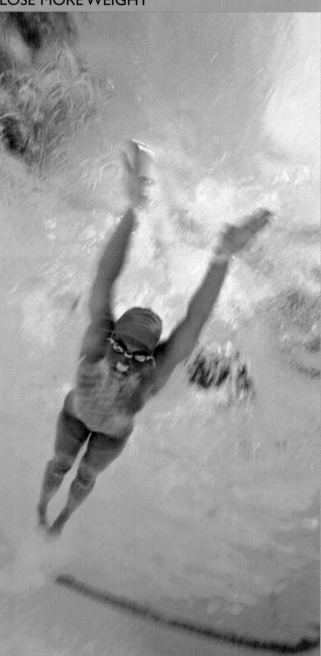

Detox in **Nine Days**

The Detox in Nine Days programme is for those who wish to detox rapidly. This programme is strict and should not be undertaken until after you have detoxed from chemicals (see pp. 34–43).

Ideally, you should choose a week when you are not working, or have minimal commitments. In any case, the first two days should be as free as possible, and for most people this means starting on a Saturday.

THE WEEK BEFORE

During the week before you plan to start the programme, read through the instructions and make a list of the things you will need. Try to borrow a juicer and food processor if you do not own these. Start off your seed sprouts (see p. 63). Read through the sections on detox supports, herbs and supplements (see pp. 74–76), and stock up on the items you plan to use, such as a skin brush, aromatherapy and massage oils, salts for hydrotherapy, and your chosen mineral and vitamin supplements.

Stock up on dietary basics, including lemons or limes to flavour your water, cold pressed olive oil, bottled still mineral water (or a new filter for your jug), and other drinks such as herbal teas (see p. 77) and dandelion tea and coffee (see pp. 74–75). You will also need to buy the food items mentioned in the dietary instructions. For a few days before you start your detox, prepare your digestive system by eating a light diet based on fruit, vegetables, rice, quinoa or millet, and chicken or fish.

DETOX **TIMETABLE**

Plan your detox timetable. Make a wall chart, if this helps, and allow time to complete the following sessions each day:

- Exercise: one yoga session (see pp. 92–93) and one brisk walk of 20–30 minutes (see p. 91).

- Meditation/relaxation/visualization: try to fit in two 20-minute sessions (see pp. 100–103).

- Skin brushing (see p. 94) or a massage, either professional or self-massage (see p. 67).

- Hydrotherapy: one session (see pp. 94–97).

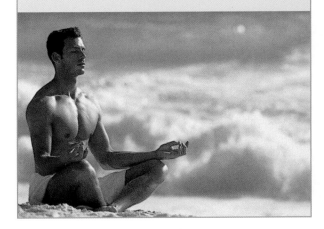

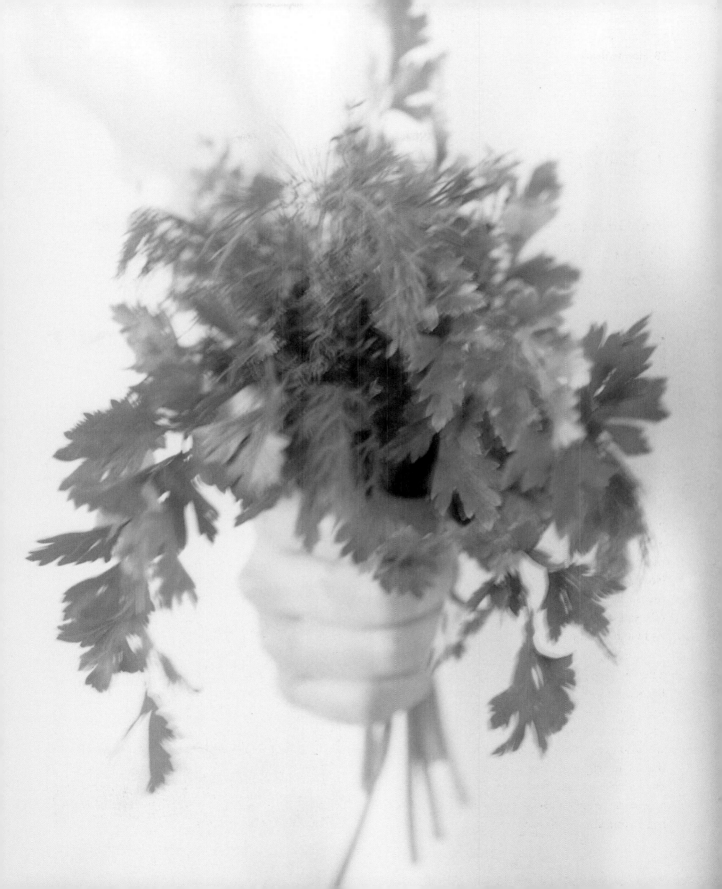

Days **one and two**

During the first two days, take plenty of rest, listen to music, read or spend time on a quiet hobby, but try to complete your detox diary schedule (see p. 58). If you are new to meditation or relaxation, you may find that your mind wanders, but just bring it gently back. If you feel sleepy, listen to your body and take some extra sleep. If your sweat smells unpleasant, take extra showers or warm (not hot) baths. Do not drive or operate machinery. Drink at least eight glasses or mugs of fluid, but not more than 15, on each of these days, and take a laxative supplement such as psyllium or linseed (see pp. 74–76) if you need to. For any withdrawal symptoms or side effects, see pp. 82–85.

SALAD DRESSINGS

Salad dressings can also be used on vegetables. Avoid commercial dressings, as these contain food additives. Use pure olive oil and lemon or lime juice, plus crushed garlic if desired, or whizz together 60–70g/2–3oz tomato juice (home-made if possible, otherwise buy a jar or carton) with half an avocado in a liquidizer and add a selection of chopped herbs such as chives, basil and parsley. For a low-calorie dressing, use live low-fat yoghurt with garlic and herbs.

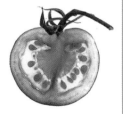

DAY 1

This is a modified fast day. You can either drink potassium broth or eat non-citrus fruit provided you do not have a candida/yeast problem (see pp. 86–87). If you choose the potassium broth (see recipe on p. 49), drink a cup every two hours. If you choose fruit, you can eat up to 1.3kg/3lb of apples, pears, grapes, peaches, apricots, mango or papaya. Have a piece of fruit every couple of hours.

DAY 2

BREAKFAST and through the morning: drink vegetable juice (see p. 69).

FOR LUNCH AND EVENING MEAL: eat either lightly steamed or stir-fried vegetables, or a large raw salad containing at least four vegetables, with a vinaigrette dressing of garlic, olive oil, lemon juice and a handful of fresh herbs. If you wish, you can also eat one piece of fruit (see day one for options). For fruit and vegetables that can aid your detox, see p. 73.

Days **three to eight**

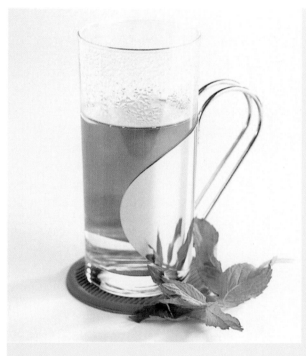

DAYS 3–8

Your diet during days 3–8 is slightly more relaxed. Continue to drink at least six to eight glasses of liquid each day, choosing from water, herb teas and vegetable juice. Take your chosen mineral, vitamin and herbal supplements (see pp. 74–76), including those with a laxative action, when needed.

ON RISING: drink one or two glasses of cold or warm water. You can add a few slices of organic lemon or lime, or their juice if non-organic.

BREAKFAST: 250–300g/8–10oz of fruit, raw or stewed, without sugar or sweetener; but avoid bananas and avocados, plus 30–60g/1–2oz of freshly shelled nuts or seeds, such as sunflower or pumpkin.

LUNCH AND EVENING MEALS are interchangeable. Choose at least four types of vegetables, including green and red/orange varieties and sprouts (see p. 78) plus a handful of fresh herbs. Eat vegetables raw, as a salad or lightly cooked by being steamed for three to four minutes or briefly stir-fried, using just enough oil to prevent them from sticking. Move them continually round the pan with a wooden spoon and do not allow them to brown. Eat when still crisp. Add a baked potato, or some rice, millet or quinoa, cooked in vegetable stock and flavoured with onion or a spice of your choice. For protein, add fish (baked or steamed), tofu, or cooked pulses such as beans or lentils. If you are still hungry, eat some fruit.

Day **nine**

Congratulations! You have nearly completed your detox. Re-score the questionnaire on pp.22–23 and check your result against your original score. You can improve your score further by following a maintenance programme.

Nine days is not long in which to alter bad habits or get rid of food cravings. For this reason, avoid bingeing on your favourite food items the day after your detox is finished. Also, the exercise plan recommended during this detox programme is really only the beginning of what should, ideally, develop into a regular and more testing programme (see pp. 90–91).

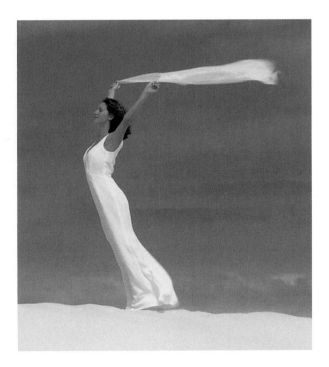

MENU FOR DAY 9

Today you will be preparing for a return to normal eating by reintroducing a wider range of foods, including wholegrains, bananas and avocado.

BREAKFAST

Porridge made with oatmeal or millet. Eat this with yoghurt (from any animal milk or soy).
Or sugar-free cornflakes or puffed rice, with soy or nut milk (see p. 55) and chopped up fruit.
Or have a grain'n'fruit smoothie: in a liquidizer; whizz together 250ml/8 fl oz (1 cup) of soy or nut milk, one banana, one tablespoonful of oatmeal or rolled oats, and berries or other fruit such as a stoned peach or fresh date, or a cored pear.

LUNCH AND EVENING MEAL

Salad or lightly cooked vegetables as on days 3–8. At one meal, have some lightly buttered wholemeal bread and some fresh fruit, and at the other meal have fish, chicken, egg(s) or a vegetarian savoury dish containing at least two different vegetable sources of protein, chosen from grains, seeds, nuts and pulses. (For further information on proteins for vegetarians, see pp. 118–119.) Have some fresh fruit and yoghurt, either made from milk or dairy-free.

GROWING YOUR OWN SPROUTS

Sprouted seeds are among the most nutritious and inexpensive foods you can eat. During germination all the nutrients needed by the young plant are mobilized from storage. The fats, starches and protein are changed into simpler chemicals that can be easily absorbed and the vitamin content increases by a huge amount. Eat them scattered on salads, added to stir-fry meals or juiced.

WHAT YOU NEED

Although you can buy commercial seed-sprouters, you may find that it is easier, and cheaper, to use glass jars. To rinse the seeds, you should cover the tops of the jars with a piece of muslin or other loosely woven fabric, attached with a rubber band. Find a warm, dark place for the seeds to germinate.

HOW TO SPROUT SEEDS

Soak the seeds in plenty of spring or filtered water; or tap water that has been boiled and cooled. Pour off the water through the muslin and rinse the seeds in fresh water; being careful to drain them well. Leave in a warm dark place, but rinse them two to three times a day until they are ready (see table). The sprouts can then be stored in a plastic bag or box for up to five days in the fridge.

Seed	Soak time (hours)	Ready to eat or store (days)	Notes
Alfalfa	6–8	5–6	Expose to light during last day of growth.
Chick peas	18	3–4	Can be cooked after two days for use in hummus, or just use them raw.
Fenugreek	6–8	3–4	Strong curry taste; use with other sprouts.
Lentils	10–15	3–5	Use whole lentils, not the split red type.
Mung beans	15	3–5	Taste bitter if exposed to light.
Mustard	6–8	4–5	Grow on damp paper towels in light and cut the green tops with scissors.
Radish	6–8	4–5	Strong taste; use with other sprouts.
Sunflower	10–15	1–2	Easily bruised, handle carefully.

The **Weekend Energizer**

Juices are a key part of the Weekend Energizer. They cleanse the body and are a great boost for a detox, being rich in minerals, vitamins and other vital nutrients.

The Weekend Energizer is an ideal detox plan for busy people who are only able to take time for themselves at the weekend, but before you start, it is best to detox, at least partly, from chemicals (see pp. 34–43). If you repeat the Weekend Energizer every one to two months and follow a maintenance programme between your Energizers, you will, over time, achieve as good a detox as with a longer programme.

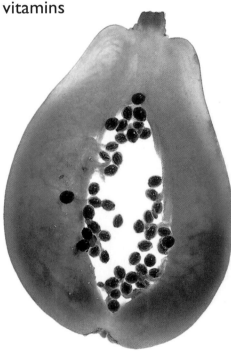

JOIN THE JUICERS THIS WEEKEND

Juicing is an essential part of the Weekend Energizer programme as it provides a high-quality boost of minerals and vitamins. Ideally, use organic produce, but if this is not possible, ensure that food is thoroughly washed, root vegetables are peeled, and the outer leaves of leafy vegetables are discarded.

VEGETABLE JUICE

Vegetable juice is a great cleanser and is an ideal way to obtain the goodness from large amounts of vegetables without having to chew your way through them. To find the juices that you like best, experiment with different proportions of vegetables and follow the instructions for your machine. You will find some starter ideas on p. 69.

If vegetable juices taste too strong you can dilute them with water.

WHY AREN'T FRUIT JUICES INCLUDED?

The downside of juicing is the loss of valuable fibre (see p. 116), which means that any sugars are absorbed too rapidly, causing fluctuations in the level of sugar in the blood (see p. 36). For this reason fruit juices are not included in the Weekend Energizer. Even some vegetable juices, such as carrot and beetroot, contain some sugar, and if you have a candida or yeast problem (see p. 86) you should mix their juice with that from other vegetables. When juices are used on an everyday basis they should be in addition to your normal fruit and vegetable intake.

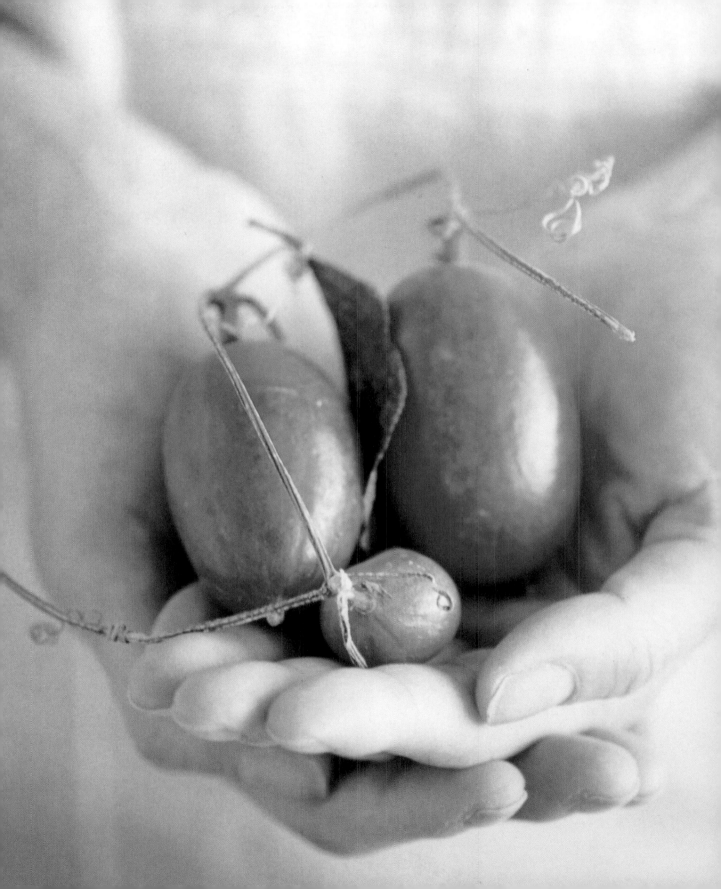

Preparing for your
Weekend Energizer

On Friday you will need to buy supplies for the weekend, including a skin brush, massage and aromatherapy oils (see pp. 94–97), if you do not already have these. During the weekend you will be eating whole fruit and plenty of vegetables, raw or lightly cooked, as well as vegetable juices.

SHOPPING LIST FOR ENERGIZER
- 0.5–1kg/1–2lb of fruit: choose your favourites, but avoid bananas.
- 3–4kg/8–10lb of salad and other vegetables. For juicing, you will need carrots, beetroot, celery and some leafy vegetables such as mustard greens, lettuce, cabbage and spinach. For your salads or lightly cooked vegetable meals it is important to include a wide variety of green, red and yellow vegetables. Read through the suggested menus on the next few pages to help you decide which vegetables you will need.
- A supply of fresh herbs.
- Still mineral water or a new filter for your jug.

FRIDAY EVENING
Eat a light, early supper around 6pm. Choose from a salad, dressed with olive oil and lemon juice, or lightly cooked vegetables. Add a baked potato or brown rice, quinoa or millet. Sprinkle with fresh herbs. Follow with fruit, plus yoghurt. Relax with a massage and have a bath or shower, followed by an early night.

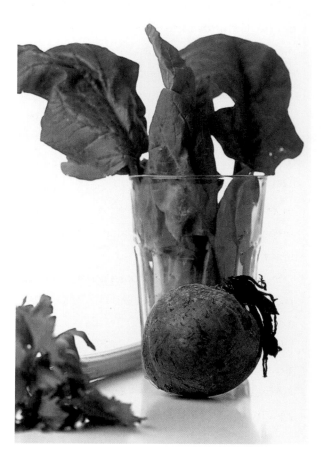

SELF **MASSAGE**

Choose a cold pressed, unrefined oil such as olive, almond, sunflower or safflower, to which your skin is not sensitive. If you are not sure, dab a little behind your ear and leave uncovered and unwashed for 24 hours. If the skin does not become red or itchy, the oil is safe to use. To 60ml/2fl oz of massage oil you can add, if you wish, a relaxing aromatherapy oil (see p. 97), or 400iu of vitamin E and 25,000iu of vitamin A. These vitamins can be obtained from supplement capsules. If you have a sensitive skin, any additives should be tested in the same way as the base oil. Warm the oil by placing the container in warm water.

Start with your legs. One at a time, gently stroke your lower legs, from the toes upwards; this aids the blood's return to the heart and stimulates the flow in your lymph vessels. Gradually make your touch firmer, kneading the calf muscle. Repeat the light touch followed by firmer pressure on your thighs and then on each arm in turn, starting with the hands and forearms.

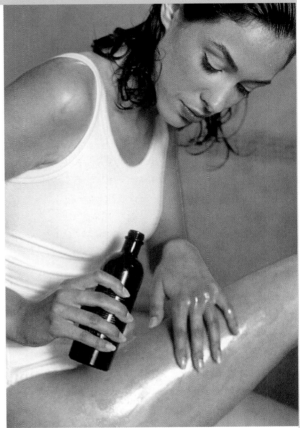

Stand up and repeat the process on your buttocks and lower back, and then on the back of your neck in a downward direction.

Lie down and gently massage your abdomen, using a circular motion in a clockwise direction.

Massage your face. Use the tips of your fingers to perform small, symmetrical slow circular movements, starting at the chin and working upwards; then stroke the skin of your forehead from the centre towards the temples. Finally, return to the chin and apply a gentle pinching act on along the edge of the jaw towards each ear.

Wrap yourself in a towel or dressing gown, and rest for a while before having a warm shower or bath.

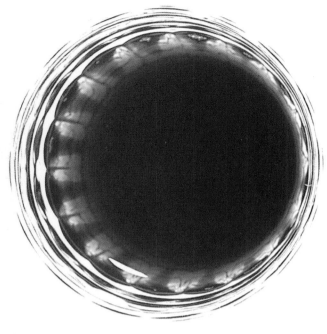

SATURDAY

On Saturday enjoy some quiet moments of relaxation as you sip one or two glasses of warm or cold water first thing in the morning. You can flavour the water with a few slices of organic lemon or lime or a few drops of juice if you cannot obtain organic fruit. Then brush your skin (see p. 94) and have a leisurely bath or shower. Dress in comfortable, loose clothes: these may need to be warmer than usual if you are feeling chilly (see p. 82). Do some gentle stretching exercises or yoga (see pp. 92–93). Unless it is very cold, have the window open for these exercises or do them in the garden.

For breakfast sip a glass of vegetable juice. If it tastes too strong, dilute it with water. During the morning, relax as much as possible. Read, listen to music, enjoy a quiet hobby and drink at least one glass of water, to which lemon or lime can be added. This is often a good time to meditate or do relaxation exercises (see p. 100).

Have a glass of vegetable juice for lunch and then go for a gentle walk lasting at least half an hour. Drink more water during the afternoon or, if you feel cold, have a warming ginger and cinnamon drink (see p. 74). Then relax or have a massage.

For your evening meal, eat at least four types of vegetable, either in a salad or lightly steamed, with a home-made dressing (see p. 60). Add a generous handful of chopped herbs. During the evening drink some more water. Before having another early night, brush your skin and have a body wrap (see p. 97) or other gentle hydrotherapy treatment.

SUNDAY

On Sunday follow the same routine as you did on Saturday but, in addition, eat one or two pieces of fruit during the afternoon. For your evening meal you can include a portion of brown rice, millet or quinoa. Eat a light dessert of one or two pieces of fruit.

MONDAY

Ease yourself back to a normal diet by eating a breakfast of two to three pieces of fruit, plus some toast and honey if you are hungry, or a grain'n'fruit smoothie (see p. 62). For lunch have a baked potato or a portion of brown rice, quinoa or millet, with a salad containing 30–60g/1–2oz of seeds or freshly shelled nuts. For your evening meal have either another salad or some lightly cooked vegetables with brown rice, quinoa or millet, and some fish or organic chicken. If you are a vegetarian, choose tofu, quorn or another protein dish (see pp.118–119).

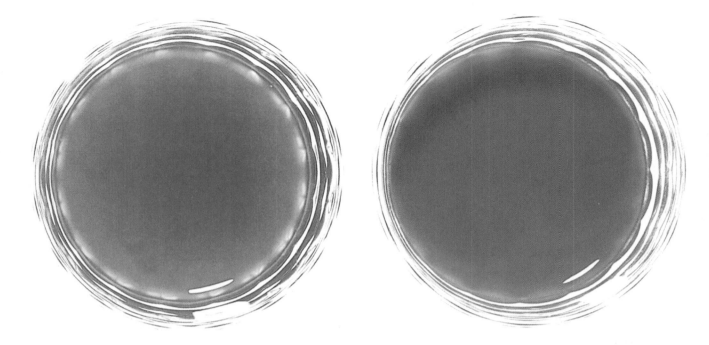

DETOX **JUICES**

Carrot, beetroot and celery are all great detox juices but, to avoid having too much sugar at once, it is best to dilute the first two with celery or other vegetable juices (see super vegetables, p. 78). Other suitable vegetables include broccoli, green leaves such as cabbage, lettuce, spring greens, turnip and beet tops, tomatoes, onions and sprouted seeds. Flavour with herbs, garlic, dried spices such as cinnamon, or hot vegetables, such as a green chilli pepper. If you like sea vegetables, pop one or two sheets into a blender with your prepared juice.

TRY THE FOLLOWING COMBINATIONS:
- Carrot and broccoli, plus a few dandelion leaves.
- Tomato, fennel and parsley.
- Carrot, celery, lettuce, coriander.
- Beetroot with sprouted seeds such as alfalfa or mung beans (see p. 63).
- Celery with a small onion and watercress.
- Carrot, beetroot, spinach and chives.
- Carrot, celery and radishes.
- Tomato, beetroot, celery and cucumber.

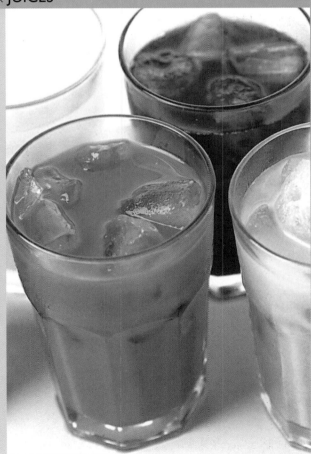

Mini-fasts and mono-diets

If you are anxious about following a longer programme, or even about the whole idea of detoxing, you may find that mini-fasting or eating a mono-diet provides a brief introduction into a detoxing lifestyle.

Mini-fasts and mono-diets can be so effective, if used regularly, that you may not need to use other programmes, or you can use them as part of a maintenance programme (see Part Three) to refresh a previous, but longer, detox programme.

A mini-fast or mono-diet can be followed for either one or two days, and you can choose a strict routine, or a gentle approach that is easily compatible with working. The brevity of the programme means that you are unlikely to develop severe side effects (see pp. 82–85), but it is important to minimize any symptoms that might arise by drinking at least six to eight glasses of water during the day. You will also benefit from having previously detoxed from, or at

least reduced, your chemical load (see pp. 34–43). Even though these programmes are so short, you can enhance their benefits by including one or more of the extra options, such as skin brushing, hydrotherapy or relaxation. Gentle exercise, preferably in the open air, is also helpful. You should seek professional advice if you wish to extend a mini-fast or mono-diet for more than two days.

PREPARATION FOR A MINI-FAST OR MONO-DIET

Read through the programmes and buy the food and other things that you will need, such as a skin brush, and massage and aromatherapy oil for the added programmes you have chosen. You should also buy still mineral water, or a new water filter, mineral and vitamins supplements (see pp. 122–123) and psyllium (see p. 76) or linseeds (see p. 75).

The night before your mini-fast or mono-diet, eat your evening meal early. This should be a light meal such as a salad or lightly cooked vegetables, with a baked potato or a portion of brown rice, quinoa or millet. This can be preceded by vegetable soup or followed by one or two pieces of fruit, raw or stewed without sweetener. Drink plenty of water during the evening, have a hydrotherapy treatment (see pp. 94–97) or a massage (see p. 67) and go to bed early.

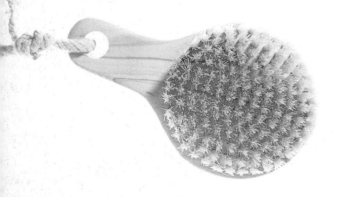

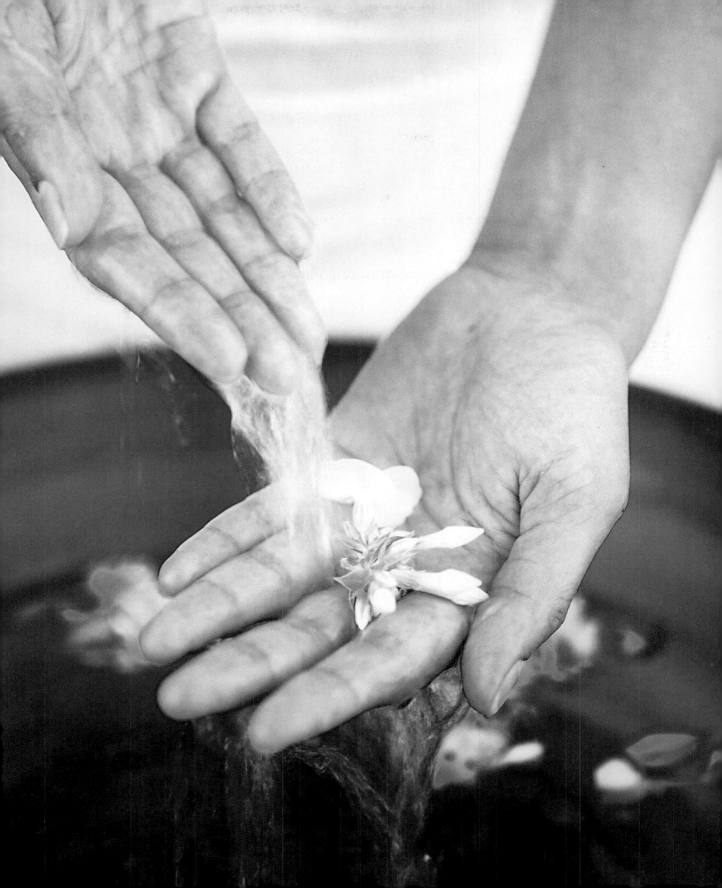

Mini-fasting

Few people used to three meals a day are happy at the idea of going without food altogether, even for a short period such as one day. However, such a fast is common when you have a dose of 'flu or a tummy upset. By not asking your body to digest food for a few hours you will enable it to catch up with any backlog of toxins.

Breakfast is so named because it breaks the overnight fast which you will have already lengthened by eating your last meal early the previous evening. This can be easily extended until midday, by just drinking water to which you can add a few slices of organic lemon or lime, or their juice if the fruit is non-organic. Alternatively, you can drink freshly made vegetable juice (see p. 69). If these options are added together, an 18–20-hour mini-fast is easily achieved, and the exercise can be repeated weekly or a couple of times a month.

Break your fast at midday or in the early afternoon with a light meal, such as a salad or lightly cooked vegetables with a baked potato, or a portion of rice, quinoa or millet, and a piece of fruit. In the evening, have more salad or lightly cooked vegetables, and add fish, poultry, without the skin, an egg or a vegetarian dish, and some fresh fruit.

An alternative approach to mini-fasting is to eat only one meal a day, and to drink plenty of water, vegetable juice or herbal tea at other times. The meal can be based on fish, or brown rice, quinoa or millet, with steamed vegetables or a salad, and some fresh fruit. Such a meal is best eaten during the middle of the afternoon.

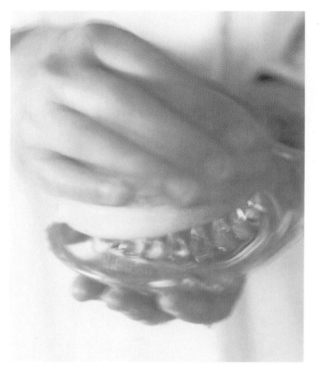

Mono-diets

Mono-diet days can be a helpful way to start detoxing, especially for people prone to hypoglycaemia (low level of sugar in the blood, see p. 36), because you can eat several single-food meals that contain starch or slow-release sugar. By only eating one type of food for one or two days, you reduce the toxic load (see p. 18) you are putting on your body. The resulting detox can be surprisingly effective.

Choose between a raw or a cooked single food diet, organic if possible. During a raw diet, you can eat up to 1½kg/3lb of one type of raw fruit or vegetable per day (see box). For a cooked food diet, you can eat 1–1.3kg/2–3lb of potatoes or up to 450g/1lb dry weight of brown rice, buckwheat, quinoa or millet. Choosing the cereal option can help to reduce blood pressure. Cook these foods in plain water, but you can dress each serving with one teaspoonful of olive oil and the juice of a lemon or lime.

FRUIT AND VEGETABLE **MONO-DIET**

For a fruit or vegetable mono-diet choose from:

Apples: help to reduce cholesterol, as they are rich in fibre (see p. 116).

Grapes: rich in potassium (see p. 123) and slow to release their sugar (see p. 117).

Pears: rich in fibre (see p. 116), vitamin C (see p. 80) and potassium (see p. 123).

Papaya: contains enzymes that aid digestion.

Carrots: can relieve wind and heartburn.

Celery: increases the production of urine, which aids detox and can help to reduce blood pressure.

AFTER YOUR MONO-DIET

At the end of your mono-diet, reintroduce a wider diet gradually as you will feel bloated if you eat a heavy meal, even after only one day's mono-diet. Eat fresh fruit for breakfast, with low-fat plain yoghurt and a little honey. For lunch have a salad with some cottage cheese or tofu and some fresh fruit. Add a baked potato or portion of rice, quinoa or millet if you are hungry. In the evening, eat a stir-fry or lightly cooked vegetables with fish, poultry (without skin), tofu or quorn. Follow with fresh or stewed fruit.

Herbs and detox **supports**

Your body may need some assistance while you follow a detox programme. This can be obtained from plants such as herbs, vegetables and fruit. In addition, you may choose to take mineral and vitamin supplements.

For thousands of years, herbs have been prepared in many ways for use as healing agents, and modern scientific research often confirms their beneficial properties. They are powerful and have to be treated with respect, but they are usually gentle as well.

Other plants are eaten every day for their nutritional value and to impart extra flavour. Many of these also have mild medicinal effects, including support for the liver, enhancement of kidney function, and promotion of relaxation. One of the most exciting recent scientific advances has been the increasing recognition of the ways that eating plants of all types can be a positive benefit to health.

TAKE **CARE**

When you use manufactured herbal preparations and the other supplements mentioned in this book, it is important to follow the manufacturer's advice regarding the dose. If you regularly take any medication, or have any medical condition, consult your doctor or healthcare professional before starting to use them. If you develop any symptoms, stop taking the preparation and seek professional advice as soon as possible.

HERBS AND SPICES WITH MEDICINAL PROPERTIES

There are several herbs and spices that can help the process of detoxing. They include the following:

Burdock acts as a mild detoxifier and can promote the production of urine and sweat.

Chamomile is most frequently taken as a relaxing tea that also aids digestion and the production of urine. As a member of the daisy family, it should be used with caution if you are allergic to other members of this family, including ragwort, which is a common cause of hayfever.

In Chinese medicine, **cinnamon bark** is used to warm and energize the body, and **ginger-root** to promote sweating and stimulate the circulation. They can be used as a warming drink, especially in the early stages of your detox. Simmer a few slices of ginger-root in 180–250ml/6–8 fl oz of water for ten minutes and then add a pinch of cinnamon. Avoid large amounts of cinnamon during pregnancy.

Dandelion is a major tonic, and good source of potassium (see p. 123). In the liver, it reduces congestion and improves the flow of bile, and in the

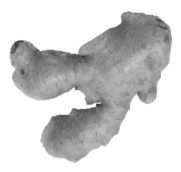

kidneys it enhances the flow of urine. Fresh, young leaves can be added to salads or made into a tea or infusion (see p. 77). You can buy dandelion tea and coffee or take the dried herb as a supplement. If you wish to make your own dandelion coffee, dry the scrubbed roots in the oven at a gentle heat. Then grind or break into small pieces and, for one day's supply, add a tablespoonful of dandelion root to 500ml/17fl oz of water in a saucepan, bring to the boil and simmer for 30 minutes. Strain before drinking, and store any leftover coffee in the fridge.

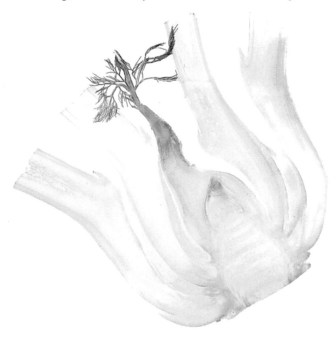

Fennel acts as a digestive aid to relieve cramps and wind. It may also stimulate appetite. Avoid high doses in pregnancy as it stimulates the womb.

Ginger decreases nausea which can sometimes arise during a detox. Make an infusion (see cinnamon, p. 74), without adding cinnamon.

Golden seal is often used as a general tonic for the liver, and to counteract sluggish digestion. It also has a laxative action. It should be avoided during pregnancy or if you have raised blood pressure.

Hops can be used before a meal as an appetite stimulant and to relieve cramps and wind. Two teaspoons of fresh hops infused for five minutes in a cup of boiling water at bedtime can relieve insomnia. Avoid if you are depressed, as it can make you feel worse. Use gloves if you gather the fresh herb, because it can cause dermatitis.

Linseeds (flaxseeds) are rich sources of omega-3 oils (see p. 121), which boost the liver, and the seeds can further aid the detox process by their laxative action. To release the oil, break down the hard seed coat in a liquidizer or coffee grinder just before you eat them, sprinkled on fruit or cereal. They can also be eaten whole, with plenty of water, as a laxative. Start with a dessertspoonful and adjust the dose to your needs.

Milk thistle or **silymarin** has been used for centuries as a liver tonic, and more recently it has been the subject of much research, confirming its role in supporting and rejuvenating the cells of the liver.

Pine bark is a source of procyanidolic oligomers (PCOs). These are powerful antioxidants and also help to reduce cholesterol levels.

Psyllium can lower cholesterol levels by up to 20 per cent in only eight weeks. The soluble fibre in psyllium attaches itself to cholesterol and other toxins in the intestine and enables them to be discharged in the stool. It is best taken at the start of a meal. To reduce your appetite, take a teaspoon of ground or powdered psyllium husks in a glass of water or juice half an hour before meals.

Rosemary eases migraines and tension headaches when taken as a tea, or as a supplement. It may also relieve exhaustion and fatigue.

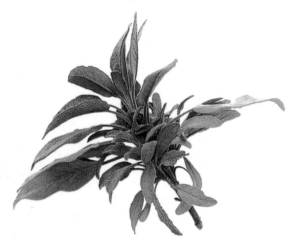

Sage infusions can act as a tonic and liver stimulant, by promoting the flow of bile. Avoid if you have epilepsy, as therapeutic doses may precipitate a fit, or if you are pregnant (culinary use is safe).

HERBAL TEAS

During a detox programme, it is best to avoid herbal teas that contain caffeine. These include mate (tea from Argentina), green and black teas, and to restrict those that contain tannin, such as mate, rose hip, yellow dock, comfrey and peppermint, which can interfere with the absorption of iron. This still leaves a wide choice of proprietary teas, including lemon balm, lime flower. linden blossom, raspberry leaf, lemon grass, chamomile and fennel.

Slippery elm is the powdered bark from this tree. One or two teaspoonfuls, taken twice a day, soothe the lining of the intestines and aid the expulsion of toxins by providing a gentle laxative action.

Turmeric is used in Chinese and Indian medicine to treat many conditions. It is the spice that gives some curries a yellow colour and it can be safely taken in liberal amounts in the diet. The active ingredient, curcumin, is a powerful antioxidant that protects the cells of the liver and stimulates bile flow.

Valerian is frequently included in herbal preparations that are sold to treat insomnia. Avoid driving or operating machinery when taking it.

Yellow dock stimulates the flow of bile and increases urine production.

HERBAL TEA RECIPE

Other medicinal and culinary herbs can also be made into herbal teas or infusions. For a pleasant drink, you can adjust the amount of herb to suit your taste, but do not exceed the amount used in the recipe below. If you are seeking a medicinal effect, use the following recipe, except for children and older people, who should have weaker infusions. If you are in doubt you should seek professional advice.

Place not more than 30g/1oz of dried herb or 75g/3oz of fresh herb in a teapot or other container with a tight lid.
Add 500ml/17fl oz of water that is just off the boil, and cover:
Leave for ten minutes then strain through a nylon sieve, and drink warm or cold.
Herbal infusions can be stored in a fridge for up to 24 hours.

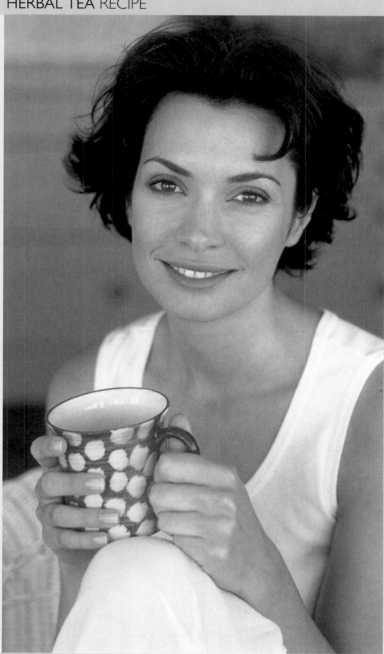

Super **vegetables**

In the West we often nibble when we feel like it, rather than sitting down to a cooked meal. As a result, it can be easy to miss out on fresh vegetables, which are stuffed with health-giving goodness and are essential in detox programmes.

Alfalfa acts as a laxative, improves the flow of urine and is a rich source of many nutrients. You can sprout it very cheaply (see p. 63) or take it as a supplement. Avoid it if you have lupus or any other auto-immune problem, because alfalfa can make these worse.

Globe artichokes promote the flow of urine, enhance liver function and help to reduce cholesterol levels in the blood. They can also relieve unpleasant breath and body odour.

Beetroot and carrot can boost the action of the liver, as they contain plenty of antioxidants. They are best eaten raw, as this slows the release of their sugars.

The cabbage family is huge and contains many of the superstars of the vegetable world. The family includes cabbage, broccoli, turnips, mustard greens, radishes, Brussels sprouts, Chinese greens and many others, each of which brings its own mix of antioxidants and nutrients to nourish your detox system. In many parts of the world, you should be able to eat one or more of its members, locally grown, preferably raw or juiced, every day.

Celery juice and extract of celery seed promote the flow of urine and can also relieve indigestion.

Garlic, onions and leeks boost the function of the liver and other parts of the immune system of the body. They also help reduce cholesterol levels.

Parsley cleans the breath after eating garlic and the other members of the onion family. In addition, it contains a number of antioxidants, and stimulates the production of urine.

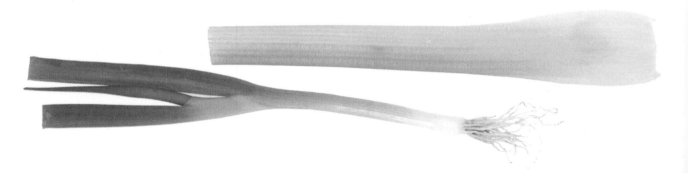

Fruit favours detoxing

Fruits, when eaten whole, are good sources of fibre and release their sugar slowly. They are, therefore, useful to control hunger when you are undertaking a detox programme.

Most types of fruit contain a particular type of sugar called fructose, which is absorbed slowly. Fructose raises the level of sugar in the blood very gently, as it is absorbed slowly and then has to be converted to glucose in the liver before the body can use it. Eating a piece of fruit 30 minutes before a meal can help to control hunger during a detox programme and this can also aid weight loss.

Apples are rich in soluble fibre, which can help to control the levels of cholesterol and sugar in the blood. They are also liver stimulants.

Apricots and peaches are rich sources of betacarotene, which is converted into vitamin A in the body. Vitamin A is essential for the liver to detox effectively.

Berries such as blackberries, raspberries, blueberries and strawberries are rich sources of fibre and antioxidants.

Grapefruit can help to reduce detox reactions. Grapefruit juice and flavonoid supplements that contain naringen (the active ingredient) can interfere with the action of certain drugs. Before you start taking them, you should check with your doctor

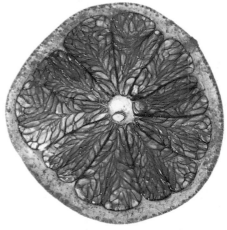

if you take regular medication, including the contraceptive pill.

Grapes are rich in antioxidants. Grapes and grape juice have long been used in mono-diets. An extract from the seeds of grapes provides procyanidolic oligomers (PCOs), which are powerful antioxidants, and it is available as a food supplement.

Kiwi fruits are rich in vitamin C. Slice off the top and eat like a boiled egg.

Papaya and pineapple contain enzymes that are helpful for digestion.

Watermelon helps detox by increasing the flow of urine.

Nutritional **supplements**

The need for mineral and vitamin supplements is controversial. Many doctors believe that we should be able to get an adequate supply of these essential nutrients by following a healthy, balanced diet.

Other doctors advocate eating as good a diet as possible and then taking modest amounts of supplements as a health insurance. There are several reasons for the latter advice:

• We often do not choose to eat the healthiest diet possible.

• Unlike compost and manure, the chemical fertilizers used on the land for the last 50 years have not been replacing a number of vital minerals such as magnesium (see p. 123) and selenium (see p. 123), so these are less plentiful for crops to take up.

• Many vitamins are lost when food is stored.

• Our detox systems are having to deal with increasing numbers of chemical toxins, and need plenty of minerals and vitamins to do this effectively.

Ideally, you should work out your individual needs with the help of a doctor who has special knowledge of nutrition or a qualified nutritional therapist. For many people, however, this is not possible and the list given opposite provides basic guidance.

NOTES AND CAUTIONS

If possible, buy natural, organic vitamins, preferably labelled as being free from yeast, lactose, starch, sugar and preservatives. It is important to follow the instructions about storage and not to exceed the recommended dose. Some minerals and vitamins are toxic in high doses, and the safe dose can be exceeded if you take supplements from more than one source. Avoid supplementing with single members of the B-vitamin family as they work together and have to be balanced. Fat-soluble vitamins (vitamins A, D, E and K) should be taken with a meal that contains fat, as this aids their absorption. If possible, take zinc last thing at night. If you have any medical condition, take medication regularly or are pregnant, check with your doctor or nutritionist before taking mineral and vitamin supplements.

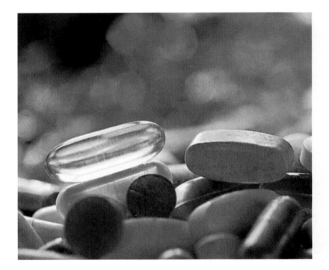

SUPPLEMENTS

Vitamin	Suggested supplementary dosage range for adults
Vitamin A	2500–5000iu
Vitamin B1	5–10mg
Vitamin B2	5–15mg
Vitamin B3	10–50mg
Vitamin B6	10–20mg
Vitamin B12	20–100mcg
Pantothenate	20–50mg
Folic acid	400–600mcg
Inosital	30–50mg
Vitamin C	200–1000mg
Vitamin E	60–400iu
Vitamin D	50–400iu
Bioflavonoids	20–100mg
Biotin	50–300mcg
Calcium	100–400mg
Magnesium	100–200mg
Iron	5–15mg
Zinc	10–20mg
Manganese	5–10mg
Copper	1–3mg
Chromium	50–100mcg
Selenium	50–100mcg
Iodine	50–100mcg
Molybdenum	50–75mcg
Boron	1mg

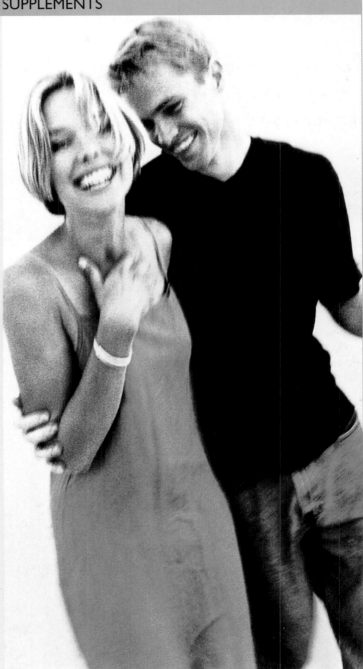

Dealing with **side effects**

As you detox, the biochemistry of your body undergoes some changes, which can result in a number of unpleasant, but harmless, symptoms. The more severe the symptoms, the more it is clear that you need to detox.

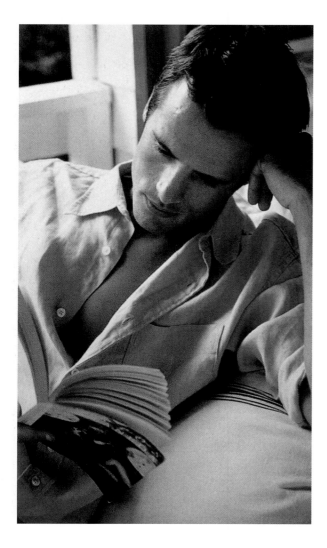

These symptoms are partly the result of your body releasing chemicals that it has been unable to deal with effectively. These chemicals are stored, often in the fatty tissue, until the body has the capacity to neutralize them. During a detox programme you withdraw from chemical stimulants and reduce the intake of other toxins, which gives your body the chance to deal with any backlog.

Fortunately, the symptoms can be lessened in a number of ways. First, before starting any other dietary restriction, stop taking non-essential chemicals such as caffeine, sugar, alcohol and drugs (see pp. 34–43), and avoid exposure to tobacco smoke. To minimize the side effects that may occur from stopping these chemicals, take some extra vitamin C and drink at least eight glasses of water a day.

Second, do not be overambitious in your choice of a detox programme. It is best to start with a programme that is not too severe, as your first detox usually produces the most symptoms.

CHILLINESS
Suddenly eating less may make you feel more sensitive to cold than usual. Do not allow yourself to be uncomfortable: wrap up in warm clothes, turn up the heating and take your drinks warm instead of cold. Warm water can be surprisingly comforting.

UNPLEASANT SWEAT AND SKIN RASHES

As your body begins to detox, it often recruits the skin as a way of eliminating unwanted toxins and you may find that your sweat smells extremely unpleasant. It is important not to suppress the sweat with antiperspirant applications, so the best remedy for unpleasant sweat is frequent bathing. Not only does this relieve the odour but it also removes the unpleasant sweat from the skin where it can be the cause of rashes. Regular skin brushing (see p. 94) can also minimize these skin reactions. Avoid perfumes and scented soaps as these simply add to your toxic load (see pp. 106–107).

COATED TONGUE AND OFFENSIVE BREATH

Coating of the tongue and offensive breath are also signs of the effectiveness of the detox. Brush your teeth regularly, use mouthwashes, such as bicarbonate of soda (one teaspoon to a glass of warm water), and be sure to drink plenty of water.

NAUSEA

Nausea can sometimes be a problem at the start of detoxing, especially if you have chosen a rapid programme for your first detox. The nausea can usually be controlled by applying firm pressure, as often as it is needed, to an acupressure point above your wrist, for up to a minute. You'll find this point between the tendons of the wrist, about 4cm/1½in on the elbow side of the wrist crease. In addition, certain herbs and spices can help to control nausea, and you may find relief if you drink a ginger infusion (see p. 74) or fennel tea.

HEADACHE

Headache is a common symptom which usually occurs during the first 48 hours of a detox programme, and is especially common when you detox from caffeine. You should avoid painkillers as your body may be more sensitive to these during a detox, but 200mg of buffered vitamin C every two hours and/or rosemary tea (see p. 77) can be helpful. Firm pressure on the acupuncture point that lies in the tissue between the thumb and index finger may also relieve headache. You will find this point by pressing gently until you notice a sensitive spot, which can then be pressed more firmly for up to a minute. Take extra rest if you can.

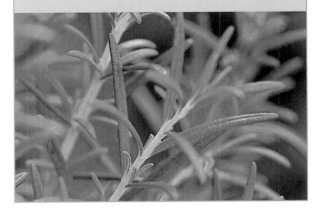

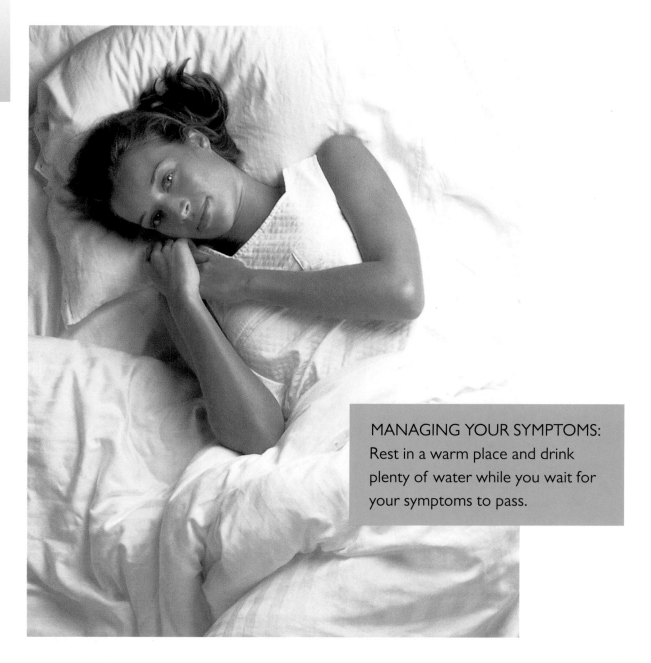

MANAGING YOUR SYMPTOMS:
Rest in a warm place and drink plenty of water while you wait for your symptoms to pass.

INSOMNIA

You may find that the dietary changes and lack of physical tiredness result in sleep disturbance. A leisurely, warm (but not hot) bath at bedtime can help to relieve the problem, especially if you add a few drops of lavender oil to the bath water. Other sleep-inducing herbs include chamomile (see p. 74), and hops (see p. 75). The relaxation techniques on pp. 100–101 can induce sleep as well as reducing any anxiety about not sleeping.

LOSS OF **CONCENTRATION**

In the early stages of a detox programme you may find that it is more difficult than usual to focus your attention on what you are doing and you may even feel drowsy. This can be the result of a sudden reduction in the amount of food you are eating, especially if you have also just suddenly reduced your intake of caffeine and sugar, or are undertaking one of the more rapid detox programmes. If this occurs, it is important to get plenty of rest. Of course, if you find your concentration is affected, you should not drive or operate any machinery.

BOWEL CHANGES

Sudden changes in diet can affect the frequency with which you empty your bowels. Fortunately, the bowel is very adaptable and will normally adjust to the changes after a few days. Constipation, which can occur at the start of a detox programme, should be avoided as far as possible, as the bowel is one of the major channels for your body to dispose of its unwanted toxins. It is important to drink plenty of fluid and if you are already prone to constipation, start to take psyllium (see p. 76) or linseed (see p. 75) sooner rather than later.

Diarrhoea is a symptom that doctors and health care professionals sometimes define in a different way from most other people. The standard diet in Western countries tends to be low in fibre, and as a result stools are small, firm and infrequent. The increased amounts of fibre recommended in detox programmes can result in stools being less firm and more frequent than usual. This is the normal stool of a diet that contains adequate fibre.

In the early stages of detox the loose watery stools of diarrhoea do occasionally occur as a result of dietary changes and the detox process. If this happens, drink extra fluid to replace what you have lost: potassium broth (see recipe, p. 49) is particularly beneficial, as potassium is lost in watery stools. If the diarrhoea lasts longer than three days you should seek professional help.

WEIGHT LOSS

For many people the prospect of losing some weight is a major incentive to undertake a detox programme. Most people lose weight in the first few days. This is largely fluid, although you will shed some fat as well once the energy stores of the liver have been used up. Some weight loss will continue during the longer detox programme, as the diet is low in fat, provided that you are not too generous with dressings that contain olive oil.

So that your body does not adapt to being given fewer calories, it is important to start an exercise programme that includes some aerobic sessions. This should be continued indefinitely to avoid putting weight on again, and starting or continuing, the socalled 'yo-yo' dieting problem (see p. 27 and p. 57). If you do not want to lose weight, make sure you eat plenty of the foods that are permitted.

Candida

If you have been told that you have a candida or yeast problem, you should avoid the few foods containing sugar or yeast that are listed in the detox programmes described in this book.

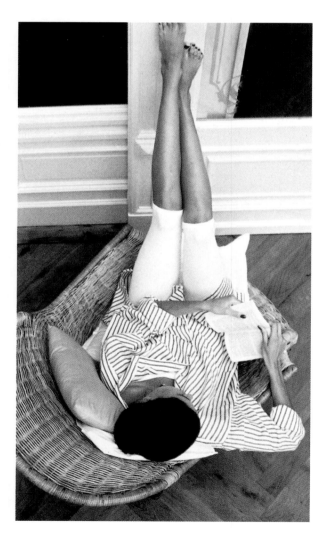

DIAGNOSIS

The diagnosis of candida or yeast problems is somewhat controversial, as the scientific proof that the intestine contains excess candida is not conclusive, and some people also become intolerant (see p. 88) to other forms of yeast, such as bakers' and brewers' yeast. All the same, many practitioners recognize that some of their patients who complain of digestive disturbance, chronic tiredness and recurrent infections with thrush (candida) and other fungi, such as athletes' foot and ringworm, do respond well to dietary changes that include removing sugar and yeast from their diet.

If you think that you could have these problems, you should obtain a professional diagnosis and guidance as to the initial treatment. This is because there are other causes for being 'tired all the time' and an accurate diagnosis is essential.

If you have had a candida problem in the past, but want to improve your health by detoxing, avoid any food that your therapist has suggested. The foods most frequently excluded are given here. It is fairly comprehensive, although you will find that most of the foods mentioned are excluded from the detox programmes anyway. If you experience symptoms when you reintroduce any of these items, you will probably need professional advice to sort out the problem.

FOODS TO AVOID IF YOU HAVE A **CANDIDA OR YEAST PROBLEM**

- Any bread product in which yeast has been used, such as bread, buns, yeasted cakes and puddings, doughnuts.

- Yeast extracts such as Marmite or Vegemite, Bovril, Oxo and other stock cubes that contain yeast.

- Any product that contains yeast. malt or 'hydrolysed vegetable protein' (read the label).

- Any fermented product such as vinegar (including most salad dressings: make your own with lemon or lime juice), soy and other fermented sauces, sour cream and other fermented dairy products, pumpernickel bread, soda bread if sour milk or cream is an ingredient, pickles and olives.

- Blue or ripe soft cheeses.

- All tomato products, but not fresh tomatoes.

- Mushrooms and quorn.

- Smoked foods such as bacon, ham, fish or cheese.

- Any fruit that is not fresh, such as dried, tinned or juiced fruits. Fresh melon is often excluded, as is over-ripe fruit.

- Any nuts, including peanuts, coconuts and their products, that have not been freshly shelled. (If you have to buy shelled nuts choose a shop with a rapid turnover of stock and store the nuts in your freezer.)

- Sugar in any form, including honey, any form of syrup, anything labelled dextrose, fructose, maltose or sucrose. Milk contains lactose and some practitioners exclude it. Yoghurt contains less lactose, but it is fermented and may be excluded for this reason.

- Dried herbs may contain moulds, so use fresh whenever possible.

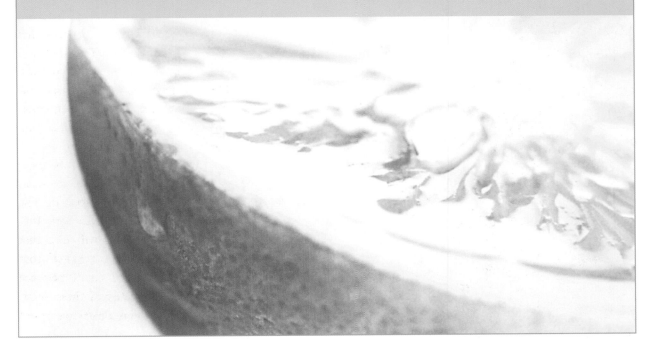

Allergies and **intolerances**

A food allergy is a reaction to a food that involves the immune system, and if your doctor has confirmed that you are allergic to any food that is suggested in this book, you should, of course, avoid it.

Food allergy is usually a lifelong condition that can be very serious as the allergy to peanuts that is reported in the news from time to time has shown. Food intolerance is different. Although it is an adverse reaction to food, the immune system is not involved in the reaction, and doctors do not, therefore, regard it as a true allergy. On the whole, people who are prone to develop food intolerance become intolerant of foods that they eat frequently. After excluding the offending food for several months they can usually eat it again without having any reaction, providing they do not have it too often.

Unfortunately, we tend to become addicted to any food to which we are intolerant, so even eating it on an occasional basis can cause problems, as it can be difficult to stop after a single portion. Many people control this tendency by continuing to exclude the food at home, but allowing themselves to eat a little when out. The reasons for this apparent addiction are uncertain, but it may be because the body produces substances called endorphins when the offending food is eaten. As endorphins are morphine-like substances the addiction is to them rather than the food.

HOW IS FOOD INTOLERANCE RELATED TO DETOX?

Food intolerance is a large topic and can be discussed only briefly here. However, many of the symptoms listed on p. 18 can be caused by food intolerance and it is likely, therefore, that a proportion of people reading this book will be intolerant of one or more foods. Diagnosing food intolerance is not easy and there is no definite test that is invariably right. Even the most commonly used tests are only about 70 per cent accurate. One of these involves removing the suspect food from the diet for a few days and then eating it again and observing whether any symptoms occur.

FOOD **INTOLERANCES**

Scientific studies have shown various degrees of intolerance to different foods, but the foods found to be most likely to cause symptoms of intolerance are:

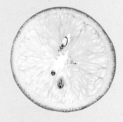

- Maize (corn)
- Milk
- Wheat
- Chocolate
- Pork
- Tea
- Oranges
- Beef
- Coffee
- Oats
- Eggs
- Sugar

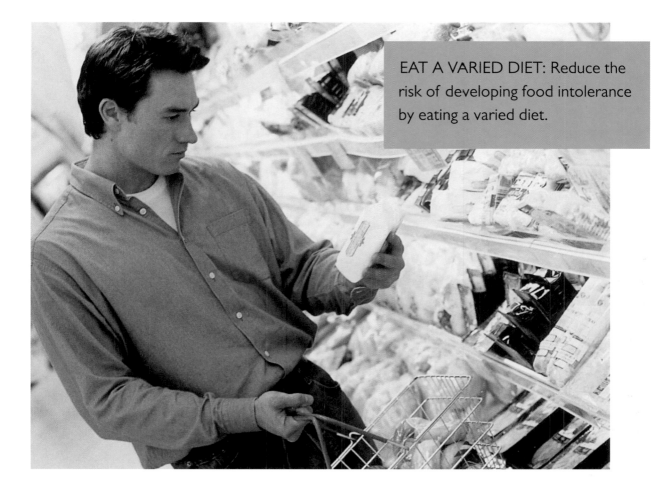

EAT A VARIED DIET: Reduce the risk of developing food intolerance by eating a varied diet.

Foods that most commonly cause food intolerance (see box) are all excluded at least in the early stages of your detox programmes. It is possible, therefore, that after following a detox programme, symptoms will come back simply because a food to which you are intolerant is re-introduced. If you think this has happened, you should seek professional guidance. If this is not possible, go back to the diet you were eating when you were symptom-free and reintroduce foods one at a time every fourth day, noting your symptoms. If you find a food that definitely seems to cause symptoms exclude it for three to four months and then eat it again. If you do not then develop symptoms, you can include the food in your diet about twice a week.

AVOIDING FOOD INTOLERANCE
The following measures may help:
- Eat a varied diet, in particular do not eat the foods listed in the box more than once a day and try to have one or two days a week when you avoid them altogether.
- Drink less tea and coffee.
- Reduce the foods that can make the wall of the gut more likely to absorb food before it is fully digested. These include highly spiced food, raw papaya and pineapple, excess alcohol, and certain drugs such as aspirin and ibuprofen.
- Eat fresh fruit and vegetables, but only when they are in season.

Exercise

Exercise boosts detox by improving the way the tissues use oxygen and dispose of waste products, eliminating waste products in sweat, making weight control easier and combating feelings of stress.

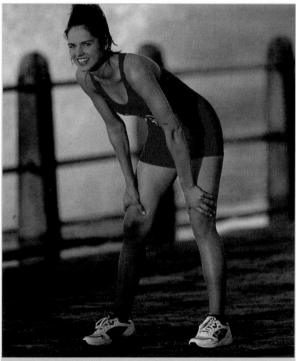

CAUTION

If you are 30+ or have any health problems at all, including being overweight, check with your doctor before starting any exercise programme. You should also consult your doctor if you experience any chest pain while exercising.

STRETCHING

Before starting exercise, it is important to stretch your muscles, as they are then less likely to be damaged. Do each of the following exercises three times.

The hamstrings are the big muscles of the back of the thigh. Stretch them by placing one foot on a chair or box, and the other about 45cm/18in away. Keeping your back straight, lean your arms on the bent knee and gradually lean forward until you feel the upper part of the straight leg being stretched. Hold for a count of 20. Repeat with the other leg.

The quadriceps muscle is on the front of each thigh. Support yourself by placing your right hand on a wall. While standing straight, bend the right knee, bringing your foot up and back, while reaching back with your left hand to grasp the right foot. Avoid straightening the left knee completely. Hold for a count of 20, and repeat on the other side.

Stretch your upper body by standing upright and clasping your hands behind your back, making sure that your elbows are straight. Pull your shoulders back, then bend forward lifting your arms above your head, elbows still straight and hands clasped. Stand straight again and, holding your clasped hands away from your buttocks and keeping your elbows straight, twist your upper body to the right and then to the left twice.

AEROBIC EXERCISE

You can exercise aerobically by running, cross-country skiing, cycling, swimming, dancing, skating and hiking. Even walking up stairs instead of taking the lift can help, but if this makes you too breathless, then start by walking down the stairs.

Pace yourself so that you can still talk, even though you are a bit breathless. If you wish to be more scientific, measure your heart rate by taking your pulse. You can feel it on the thumb side of your wrist about 2½–5cm/1–2in from the skin crease at the wrist. Count the beats for ten seconds and multiply by six.

Aim for a heart rate between 70 and 80 per cent of the maximum for your age (see table, right). If you need to lose weight, you are likely to achieve the greatest loss if you aim for about 60 per cent of your maximum heart rate and exercise for 45–60 minutes (rather than for shorter periods) about three to five times a week.

GUIDE TO **HEART RATES**

Age	70–80 per cent of max rate	60 per cent of max rate
20	140–160	120
30	133–152	114
40	126–144	108
50	119–136	102
60	112–128	96
70	105–120	90

HOW MUCH IS ENOUGH?

Spend five to ten minutes doing warm up stretching exercises. If you are very unfit, start with five minutes exercise and build up gradually to about 30 minutes. If you are still tired an hour after exercise you should do less and build it up gently.

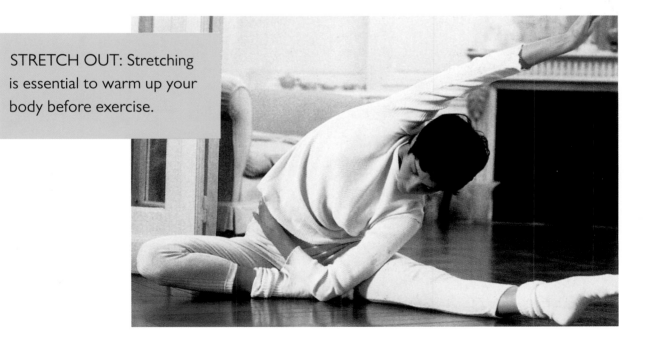

STRETCH OUT: Stretching is essential to warm up your body before exercise.

Yoga

Yoga is a gentle exercise that can aid the discharge of waste. Its practice is peaceful and enhances calm. To experience the benefits of yoga fully you will need to attend classes, but a few exercises are given here to help with detox.

If you have any health problems, especially with your back or heart, or are pregnant, you should obtain your doctor's agreement, and find a teacher who is also a qualified yoga therapist.

ALTERNATE NOSTRIL BREATHING

Alternate nostril breathing helps to empty your lungs thoroughly and maximize their detox function. It is also extremely relaxing. Sit upright in a chair, or cross-

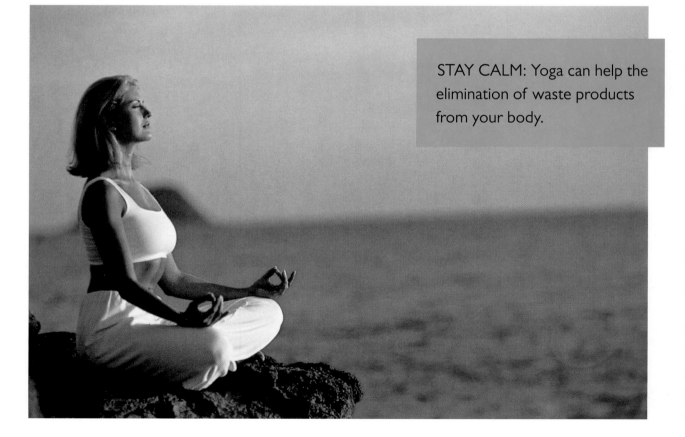

STAY CALM: Yoga can help the elimination of waste products from your body.

SALUTE TO THE **SUN**

Salute to the sun is a traditional exercise that stretches most muscles, and can help to make you more flexible. You may be rather awkward at first, but with practice it will become easier. Repeat the exercise for an even number of cycles, with a 30-second rest between them, then relax for a few minutes.

1   Stand erect with your feet together. Place your hands, palms together in front of your chest in the 'prayer' position.

2   As you inhale again, raise your hands above your head. Lean back with the palms facing up.

3   Breathe out as you bend forward as far as you can, keeping your knees straight. With practice, you may be able to rest the palms of your hands on the floor beside your feet.

4   As you inhale, bend your knees and place (or keep) the palms of your hands beside your feet. Take your right leg back and rest the knee on the floor. Look forward.

5   Breathe out as you lift the knee from the floor, place your left leg beside the right leg, and straighten them: so you are supported on your hands and toes.

6   Breathe in as you place both knees on the floor, rest your buttocks on your heels and lower your forehead to the floor. Breathe out.

7   Without inhaling, move forward so that your knees, chest and forehead, but not your abdomen, are on the floor. Then breathe in, pushing up with your arms, so that you are supported on your hands and toes again, but this time look up so that your back is concave.

8   Breathe out as you push your buttocks up, and make a triangle with the floor, keeping your heels as near the floor as you can.

9   As you inhale, bend your knees and rest your buttocks on your heels (as in 6). Breathe out.

10 As you breathe in, bring your right knee up, placing your right foot between your hands.

11 Place your left foot beside your right foot as you breathe out. Straighten your legs, but keep your hands near the floor (as in 3).

12 As you inhale, stand erect and rest briefly. Repeat the cycle putting your left leg back as in 4 and left knee up first in 10.

legged on the floor. Close your eyes and block the right nostril with your right thumb. Breathe out through your left nostril, then breathe in to a count of four, and hold to a count of 16. Using your fourth and fifth fingers, block the left nostril and release the right nostril. Breathe out to a count of eight. Repeat the exercise, this time breathing in through the right nostril. You should stop and rest if you become at all uncomfortable.

Hydrotherapy

Water, steam and ice can all be used for healing, but you do not have to visit an expensive spa to make use of water to enhance your detox programme. Simple home treatments can boost your programme.

Water has been used for cleansing and healing for thousands of years. Recent scientific experiments have shown that taking cold showers regularly can result in fewer colds. Programmes that gradually increase the body's exposure to cool and then cold water have resulted in:

- Improved energy even in those who have chronic fatigue syndrome.

- Improved fertility by enhancing the production of sex hormones.

- Better circulation for people who normally have cold hands and feet.

- Relief from menopausal symptoms.

You can obtain the benefit of hydrotherapy techniques by consulting a practitioner, but the following simple home treatments can enhance your detox programme.

SKIN BRUSHING

Skin brushing is a good exercise to wake you up in the morning and to stimulate your circulation before you take a shower. You will need to buy a natural bristle brush, bath mitt or loofah, and to get up in time to allow five to ten minutes for brushing your skin in a warm room. When brushing your skin, use light pressure and a continuous circular motion and always move towards the heart. Try to cover all the skin except, in women, the breasts.

How to Brush your Skin

Starting in a sitting position, brush the sole of one foot and, moving upwards, brush the top of the foot, ankle and lower leg. Repeat on the other side. Then stand to brush the upper legs, including the back of each leg, and then the buttocks and back. If you cannot reach all of your back, rub it briskly with a dry towel.

Next brush one hand, and move up the arm making sure that you brush all the skin. Repeat with the other arm. Gently brush the abdomen, in a clockwise direction. Finally brush your neck and upper chest, this time in a downward direction, towards the heart. Have a shower and moisturize your skin.

HYDROTHERAPY WITH A SHOWER

Most modern showers allow you to vary the jet of water you are using as well as the temperature of the water. By also varying the amount of time you spend in a shower, you have an easy access to a wide range of home hydrotherapy treatments.

TAKE THE PLUNGE: Hydrotherapy is an enjoyable way to boost your detox, improve your skin and ward off infection.

Hot Showers

Hot showers can relax you, and washing in a hot shower is the best way to clean your skin, but don't spend longer than five minutes in a hot shower, as this can be enervating. Always finish with a cold or cool shower when you want to boost the circulation to your skin and improve its tone. By constricting the circulation to the skin, cold showers initially give you a sensation of inner warmth. This constriction allows certain chemicals to accumulate in the skin. These then act to dilate the blood vessels again so that your skin feels warm and glowing and the detox function of your skin is enhanced.

Neutral Showers

A shower that feels neither hot nor cold is described as neutral. Neutral showers can be restful, and you may find that a neutral shower at bedtime helps you to relax and sleep well.

Alternating Showers

Alternate hot and cold showers are also relaxing and stimulate the circulation. In addition, they cleanse the skin of sweat very effectively. Start with a warm shower, and increase the heat until it feels quite hot. Then switch quickly to a cold shower for about 15 seconds before going back to a hot shower. You can

SALT MASSAGE BATH

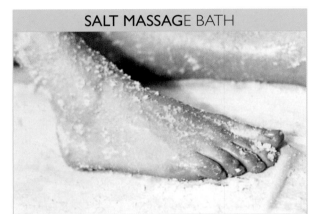

Run a warm bath. Place a handful of sea salt in a bowl and add a little water to make a thick paste and massage this into your skin, in the sequence suggested for skin brushing (see p. 94). Then soak for ten minutes or so in the bath, pat yourself dry and go to bed. Be sure to have water at hand during the night, as you are likely to sweat quite profusely when you first use this treatment. In the morning have a warm shower and apply a skin moisturizer.

CAUTION

Avoid both types of salt bath if you have any condition in which the skin is broken or weeping, or if you are feeling tired or weak. Check with your doctor first if you have a heart condition, high blood pressure or diabetes.

repeat this several times if you wish. Initially you may prefer to alternate the temperature between warm and tepid, and gradually increase the temperature difference as you become used to the therapy. You can also vary the pressure of the water to obtain the effects that you find most helpful.

HYDROTHERAPY IN YOUR BATH

An Epsom salts bath or sea salt massage bath increases sweating, which boosts your detox programme. One treatment can be repeated once a week during a detox programme, but once a month is sufficient at other times.

Epsom Salts Bath

Buy Epsom salts from a pharmacy: for each bath you will need between 250–450g/½–1lb, plus 100g/3oz of sea salt. Run a bath that is comfortably warm, add the salts and dissolve them. Lie in the bath for between ten and 20 minutes, topping up the water if you become chilled. Get out of the bath carefully, as you may feel a little light-headed, wrap yourself in several large towels and go to bed, making sure that you have plenty of water to hand, in case you become thirsty. In the morning have a warm shower or bath and apply a skin moisturizer. You will need to wash the towels before using them again, as you are likely to sweat profusely during your sleep.

AROMATHERAPY IN YOUR BATH

Essential oils can be added to your bath, but before using them it is important to check that your skin is not sensitive to them. Apply a little behind the ear, and leave unwashed for 24 hours. The oil is safe to use if the skin has not reddened or become itchy, but

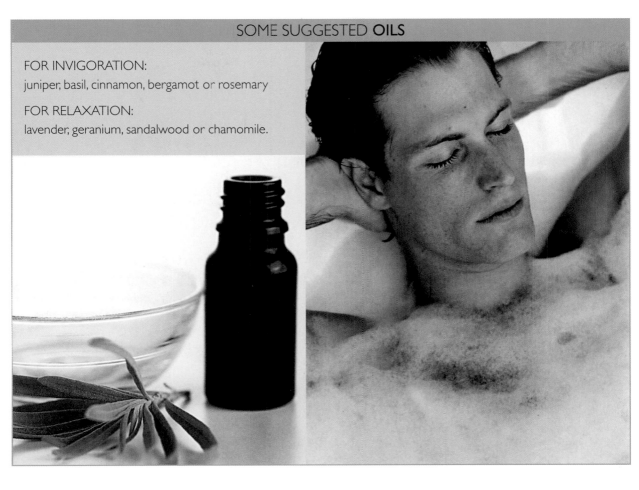

SOME SUGGESTED **OILS**

FOR INVIGORATION:
juniper, basil, cinnamon, bergamot or rosemary

FOR RELAXATION:
lavender, geranium, sandalwood or chamomile.

sensitivity may develop with frequent use of the same oil. Run your bath, using tepid water for invigoration or hot water for relaxation. Add about ten drops of the essential oils when the bath is nearly ready; then enjoy a relaxing soak.

HYDROTHERAPY BY APPLICATION

A trunk wrap can be applied without help from another person. This aids detoxing by promoting perspiration. Fold a large thick towel so that it is wide enough to cover the area from your armpits to your navel and long enough to wrap round you with some overlap. Place it on a flat surface, such as on your bed. Measure a piece of cotton material that is at least 2.5cm/1in narrower than the towel, and is long enough to go round you in a single layer without any overlap.

Dip the material in cold water, wring it out so that it is damp but not dripping, and place it in the centre of the towel. Lie on top and wrap the cotton material round you, followed by the towel, keeping them in position with large safety pins. Wrap yourself in a blanket and relax for three hours, or longer if you have the time. If you do not warm up within five minutes, take off the pack, dry yourself briskly, and repeat the exercise another day, wringing out the cotton material more thoroughly. Always wash the cotton material between applications as it will have absorbed discharged toxic waste.

Detoxing **your mind**

Most of us seem to be constantly juggling with too many commitments and too little time. As well as concentrating on your physical health during a detox programme, you can benefit from practising some mental detox exercises.

These exercises can help you to achieve a state of calmness, which can also make a contribution to improving your general physical health and well-being. In particular, regular practice may help make your sleep more refreshing, ease digestive symptoms, reduce stress on your heart by reducing your blood pressure and slowing the rate of your heart beat, and even help your immune system to ward off infection. Finally, calm people are more likely to work effectively and are more likely to be able to rid themselves of chemical addiction (see pp. 34–43), when this is necessary.

In the next few pages you will find some suggestions on relaxation, meditation and visualization. These techniques are not learned instantly, but with a little practice you will be able to do the exercises in many places, such as on a commuter train, for a few minutes at lunch time or in your bath, as well as during regular sessions at home. Obviously, these exercises are NOT appropriate while you are driving or operating machinery. At first you will probably find that your mind wanders: this is normal and should not cause you distress or irritation. Just be patient: tranquillity will come!

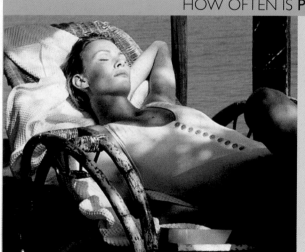

HOW OFTEN IS **PRACTICE NEEDED?**

Try to spend 10–20 minutes practising relaxation once a day, or twice if your stress levels are high. Mental detox exercises can be particularly beneficial after your yoga exercises (see pp. 92–93). At first, you are likely to spend most of the time just trying to become relaxed, but with regular practice it will become much easier, and you will find that you are spending more time simply being calm and still.

Relaxation

Changes in medical thinking mean that the close relationship between the psychological and the physical aspects of the nervous and immune systems is now recognized. Relaxation allows you to release both mental and physical tension.

As a result, you save energy, and your muscles will feel less fatigued; thus your liver and digestive system will be able to function more effectively, enhancing the detox process.

HOW CAN RELAXATION BE ACHIEVED?

There are many techniques for relaxing. Some have been practised for several centuries, but new ones are being developed all the time. Some of these, such as autogenic and biofeedback techniques are best learned with an instructor; others need special equipment (see box), but for the simple home relaxation method described below, all you will require is patience, a warm quiet room and loose comfortable clothes.

SIMPLE HOME RELAXATION

- Lie on your back on a firm, comfortable surface, with your legs straight and slightly apart, and your arms a few inches away from your body, palms upward. This relaxation technique involves tightening different muscle groups for about five seconds then relaxing for about five seconds before moving on to follow the same process with the next group of muscles.

- Extend your right foot as far as possible, curling your toes. Hold and release. Then pull your foot up as far as you can. Hold and release. Repeat on the left.

- Pull your right kneecap upwards. Hold and release. Press your leg down as hard as you can. Hold and release. Repeat on the left.

- Breathe in deeply through your mouth, hold your breath for a few seconds, then gently expel it through your nose. Spend a minute or so concentrating on the heavy feeling in your legs.

FLOTATION **THERAPY**

Weightlessness in a calm place is an ideal way to relax if you have the opportunity to use a flotation tank, in which the water is highly salted. rather like that of the Dead Sea. As a result, the weight of your body is supported so that you can lie in a totally relaxed position. The air surrounding the tank is air-conditioned, so that the atmosphere is not hot and sticky. You can choose to lie in the dark or in subdued light, and in some tanks. you may have the option of soft music.

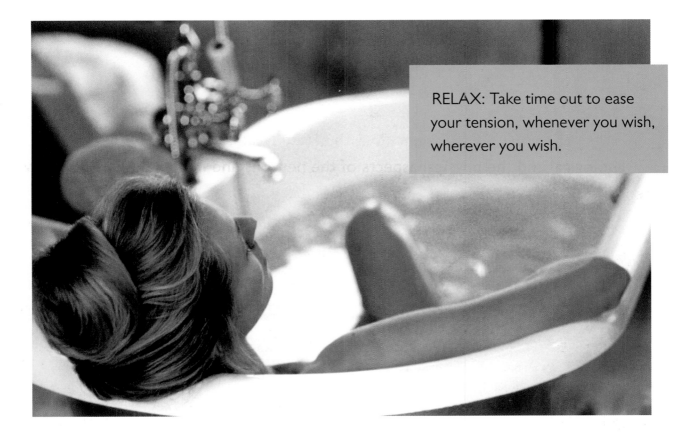

RELAX: Take time out to ease your tension, whenever you wish, wherever you wish.

- Make a fist with your right hand. Hold and release. Stretch your fingers out as far apart as possible. Hold and release. Repeat on the left.

- Bring your right hand up to your right shoulder, and tense the arm muscles. Hold and release. Push your right arm down into the surface that you are lying on. Hold and release. Repeat on the left.

- Bring your right shoulder up to your right ear. Hold and release. Push your shoulder down into the surface you are lying on. Hold and release. Repeat on the left. Breathe in deeply through your mouth, and hold it for a few seconds then gently expel it through your nose. Concentrate on your arms; feel how heavy they are.

- Tense your buttocks. Hold and release.

- Tense your abdominal muscles. Hold and release.

- Follow the same tensing and releasing routine for the muscles of your face. If you wear contact lenses, you should make sure you avoid screwing up your eyes too tightly.

- Lie quite still with all your muscles relaxed. You may find that some of them tighten again, especially those of your jaw and neck, without your consciously making them tight. Don't worry, just relax again, consciously dropping your jaw so that your teeth are not touching. You will feel as if you are smiling gently.

Meditation & visualization

Meditation techniques have been encouraged by most great religions, and many people find them beneficial. However, other people find that visualization provides a more personal approach to mental detox.

During meditation, the body is still and the attention is focused. In this state of calm alertness the electrical waves in the brain are changed, and any imbalance between the sides of the brain is removed. As a result, stress symptoms, such as sleep and digestive disorders are reduced, the heart beats more slowly, blood pressure is reduced, and detoxing is enhanced. Meditation is an ideal aid to giving up chemical addictions such as alcohol and use of tobacco.

In general, you will need to learn how to relax before you can meditate, and some people start their meditation session by formal relaxation (see pp. 100–101). For meditation, you may want to choose something to focus on. This can be a candle, an object of spiritual significance or a colour. You can choose to use a real object by gazing at it for a time, and then closing the eyes, so that the object is seen in the imagination, or simply use your imagination from the start.

Some people choose a meaningful phrase or idea, or a sound. The latter, known as a mantra in the Eastern tradition, is heard in the mind, and helps to drown out any intruding thoughts.

Worry beads, rosary beads or other objects that can be moved in the hands use touch as a point of focus, and have been employed by many people over hundreds of years.

HOW TO **MEDITATE**

- Choose a position that is comfortable for you.

- Spend a little time relaxing.

- Focus on your chosen object and gently close your eyes.

- If your attention wanders, bring it quietly back: almost everyone has this problem at first, and it can return at a later time. The important thing is not to lose your composure; just restore your concentration with as little disturbance as possible. Practise every day, twice daily if possible, for 10–20 minutes or longer.

VISUALIZATION

Once you have been practising relaxation and meditation for a while, you may wish to include visualization. This can help you achieve changes in your life. The technique includes 'seeing' your body putting right anything that has gone wrong inside itself. It has even been used by conventional doctors as a type of therapy, complementary to conventional treatment, for treating a number of illnesses including those that are life-threatening, such as cancer and AIDS.

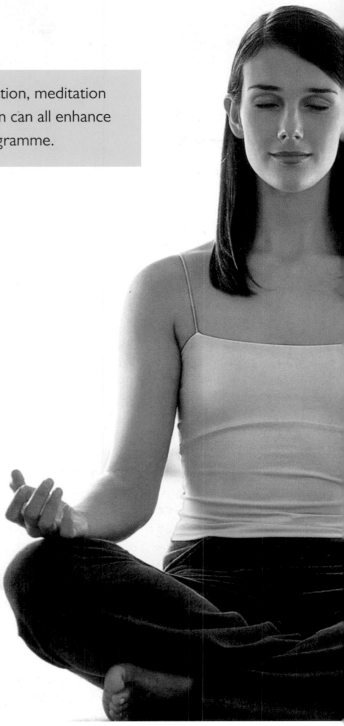

FOCUS: Relaxation, meditation and visualization can all enhance your detox programme.

Once you have relaxed, imagine yourself somewhere safe and pleasant. If you use the same image each time, you will find that you can opt out of tense situations for a few minutes by visiting your 'safe haven'. This is your own safe place where you can visualize your problems and their resolution.

External visualization allows you to 'see' yourself dealing competently with the problems that normally trouble you. This can help you to deal with past events that have left lingering, unhappy memories and to change your life by becoming more assertive and achieving what you want by gaining insight into your own condition.

Use internal visualization to imagine healing.

Physical stress can be overcome by visualizing your heart beating more slowly, your breathing calmer and your muscles relaxed. Imagine that your brain becomes still, rather than a cause of anxiety or fear. If you have been ill visualize your body healing itself.

CAUTION

Some visualizations can trigger physical symptoms. For example, visualizing a field of hay or flowers could cause hay fever or even asthma. If you suffer from respiratory problems of any type, it is best to consult your doctor before using this technique.

Detox your **environment**

You may believe that you are safe from harmful chemicals in your home and that in your work environment the law protects you. But you are likely to be wrong on both counts.

Recent reports suggest that we may be exposed to several hundred pollutants in a normal house or office. These include dust, smoke and airborne bacteria, as well as the paints, cleaners, dyes, glues, sprays, pesticides and solvents that are used every day.

The Environmental Protection Agency in the United States has estimated that indoor air pollutants may cause thousands of deaths from cancer in the US. The Agency has also reported that 'Indoor air pollution in residences (and) offices ... is ... one of the most serious potential environmental risks to health.'

Many of these pollutants can enter the body by being inhaled, absorbed through the skin, or by being eaten in contaminated food. The dietary detox programmes in this book can be enhanced if you detox your environment, and their benefits prolonged by adopting a lo-tox lifestyle.

FRIENDLY **PLANTS**

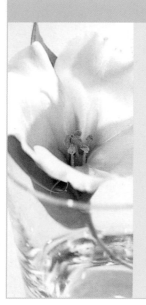

In the 1980s NASA scientists found that certain plants can remove some of the toxic chemicals that occur frequently in the modern home, such as formaldehyde, benzene, trichoroethylene and ammonia.

The plants include:
- Areca palm (*Dypis lutescens*)
- Lady palm (*Rhapis excelsa*)
- Bamboo palm (*Chamaedorea seifrizii*)
- Rubber plant (*Ficus elastica* 'Robusta')
- Spider plant (*Chlorophytum elatum vittatum*)
- Ivy (*Hedera helix*)
- Dwarf date palm (*Phoenix roebelenii*)
- Golden pothos (*Epipremnum aureum*)

Another friendly plant is the cactus (*Cereus peruvianus*), which, when placed near to television and computer screens, appears to be able to absorb some of the electromagnetic emissions.

CLEAN AIR: Green plants help to reduce greenhouse gases and absorb chemical pollutants.

Detox your **house**

In the United Kingdom, the Building Research Establishment recommends that, to minimize the effects of pollutants in the air, houses should have a complete air change every two hours.

The simplest and most effective way of reducing airborne indoor pollutants is to keep your house well aired, as it has been shown that indoor pollution is worse than that out of doors. Open all the windows for 15 minutes twice a day, and use exhaust fans when you are in the kitchen and bathroom. The air outside the house is generally drier than that inside, especially if the house is well insulated. Sweat, bathing, washing machines and cooking all contribute to the amount of water in a house, and damp air increases the chances of moulds forming, as well as being preferred by dust mites.

INDOOR CHEMICALS

Harmful chemicals are most likely to be emitted from the newest buildings and furnishings, but chemical treatments for wood rot and infestations of woodworm and other wood-boring insects can be a problem in older properties after renovation. Whenever possible, try to choose non-toxic building materials and furniture, as new paint, carpets, furniture coverings and curtains can all release toxic solvents, as can the pressed wood and fibreboard used in the fabrication of most modern furniture and built-in cupboards. Choose solid wood furniture or seal composite bonded materials with a low-toxicity sealant. Avoid carpets treated with fungicides and permanent stain-resistant chemicals. Always hang new or recently dry-cleaned clothes in the open before placing them in your wardrobe. Avoid fabric softeners, air fresheners and toilet blocks, which can all increase chemical pollution. Redecorate your house during the summer months when the heat accelerates the release of solvents and it is easier to keep the house well aired. Use water-based paints whenever possible.

COOKING AND HEATING

Cooking produces water vapour and releases food chemicals, some of which can cause asthma in sensitive people. You can minimize these problems by using a cooker hood and extractor fan, especially if you cook with gas. Gas boilers and fires should be professionally installed and regularly serviced. Solid-fuel stoves also contribute to airborne pollution, but this can be minimized by ensuring that chimneys and flues are kept clean. Wood for wood-burning stoves is another source of moulds.

SCENTS AND PERFUMES

'Chemical odour pollution', as it has been called, is becoming an increasing problem for people who are chemically sensitive and places an extra strain on everyone's detox systems. Keeping your use of perfumes, sprays and aerosols to a minimum can

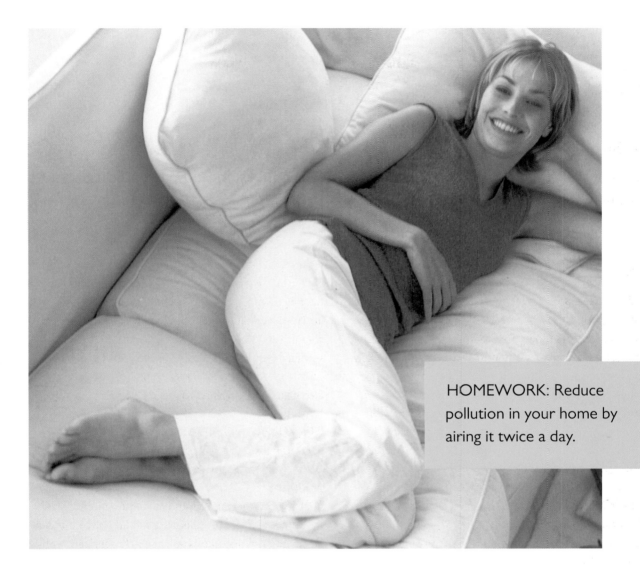

HOMEWORK: Reduce pollution in your home by airing it twice a day.

make a substantial difference to the amount of work your detox system has to perform.

DETOX THE GARDEN
Reduce your use of garden pesticides, as they add to your 'total load' (see p. 18) of pollutants, and many contain chemicals that can threaten your health. Do not wear outdoor shoes inside – they bring in pesticides and other chemicals from the garden and the street.

CIGARETTE AND TOBACCO SMOKE
You now have a right to complain about tobacco smoke in public places, and it is best to keep it out of your house, especially if you have young children. If your workplace has a special room set aside for smokers, it should have an extractor fan that continues to work after the room has been vacated. The management should also ensure that air from this room does not enter the air-conditioning system, and is not allowed to drift into other rooms or corridors.

Lo-tox **cleaning**

You will not obtain the maximum benefit from a detox programme unless you reduce the chemical pollution that creeps into your house disguised as cleaning agents.

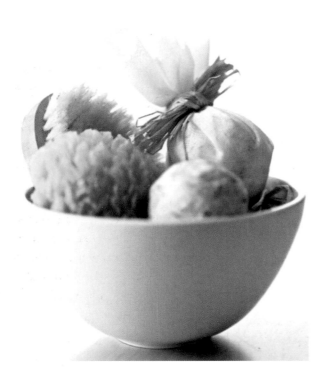

Modern polishes, detergents and the vast range of cleaning agents now available often contain volatile organic compounds (VOCs) which can be toxic and will often irritate the membranes of the nose and throat. Fortunately, there are a number of new 'green' products coming onto the market, which are less toxic. There are also some old-fashioned, and usually cheaper, alternatives that can be employed:

- Water containing sodium bicarbonate or borax is mildly disinfectant and can be used for many cleaning jobs such as washing the fridge or freezer. Use very hot water with borax to clean the toilet, or use tea tree essential oil as a stronger disinfectant.

- Dry sodium bicarbonate powder in a small glass jar with holes punched in the lid will kill smells in a fridge, cupboard or room. Carpet smells can be removed by sprinkling dry sodium bicarbonate on the carpet and vacuuming or brushing it up a couple of hours later.

- Dry sodium bicarbonate or borax placed in a dustbin or wastebin will clear smells. They can also be used on a damp brush to clean mould from tiles or grouting.

- Clean a drain by dropping a tablespoonful of washing soda on the grating and pouring down very hot or boiling water.

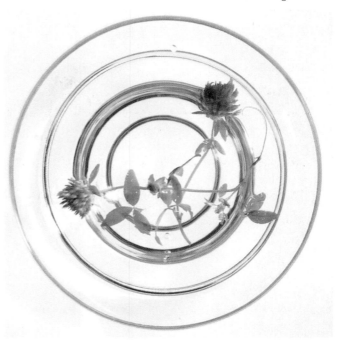

- Clean windows, mirrors and tiles by spraying on a mixture of half water and half white, distilled vinegar, and polish with a dry cloth. The same mixture can be used to de-scale a kettle: bring to the boil, leave overnight, rinse well, then fill the kettle with clean water and bring to the boil again and discard the water before using the kettle to heat water that you will be drinking.

- To remove stains from dishes or chopping boards scrub them with salt, plus a little lemon if you wish. Pure beeswax polish is usually prepared in lo-tox solvents that disperse quickly after use.

- To avoid using powerful chemical cleaners on your oven, try to clean it regularly while it is still warm, using sodium bicarbonate in hot water (one tablespoonful to 300ml/10fl oz of water).

ELECTROMAGNETIC POLLUTION

Life without electricity is hard to imagine, at least in the Western world. All electrical appliances give off electromagnetic energy, although it is at a low level for household appliances. All the same, there are researchers who believe that this energy may affect health. Possible problems include insomnia, alterations in brain function, raised blood pressure and maybe other rather ill-defined problems, such as headaches or nausea, or simply not feeling well. There are certainly some people, especially those who are more sensitive to chemicals than most people, who do seem to be particularly sensitive to electromagnetic energy.

Pre-heating your bed with an electric blanket is safe. However, couples who sleep with an electric over-blanket switched on seem more likely to suffer miscarriages or have smaller babies than those who do not. Excessive use of mobile phones should probably be avoided while their safety is further assessed.

ELECTROMAGNETIC **ENERGY**

Avoiding unnecessary exposure to electromagnetic energy seems a sensible precaution. One way is to keep appliances switched off when they are not in use. Avoid sleeping in a room with a computer or television still running or on standby. In addition to cactus plants (see p. 104), quartz crystals have the reputation of absorbing this energy. Some people keep both near to the television or computer screen, and 'rebalance' the quartz by washing it daily, under running water and drying it, if possible, in the sun.

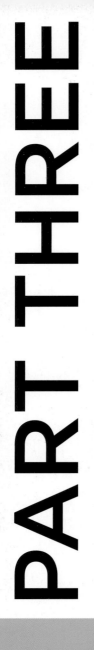

PART THREE

Stay detoxed! Choose a lo-tox lifestyle

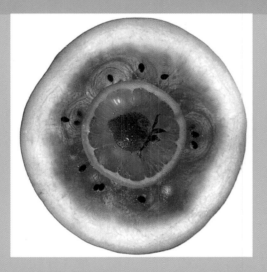

Take your detox further with a lo-tox maintenance programme.

Lo-tox **maintenance**

Once you have completed your detox programme you should feel more energetic, yet calmer and have fewer symptoms. Unfortunately, you may lose these benefits unless you 'top up' your detox from time to time.

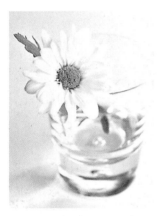

If you have not already done so, score the questionnaire (see pp. 22–23) again and compare it with the one you did before starting to detox. Now you need to plan how best to maintain this improvement with as little effort as possible.

Detoxing your environment is the foundation of a lo-tox lifestyle. A number of the suggestions that were mentioned on pp. 104–109 should be introduced to your home over a period of time, as you renew your furniture, soft furnishings and redecorate. Detoxing your workplace and general environment, such as reducing industrial and transport pollution, may also take time and will probably require patient lobbying.

Your long-term lo-tox maintenance should include all the aspects of your first detox. This means that you should include each of the following:

Refresher detoxes: How often? Which plan?

Bodywork: Programmes to keep fit and supple.

Detoxing your mind: To make the most of your work and recreation.

Eating well: Plan the most nutritious diet you can, including plenty of fresh fruit and vegetables. Eat organic when possible, but it is more important to eat plenty even if it is not organic.

REFRESHER DETOXES

Once you have taken the plunge and followed a detox programme you will find that it is relatively easy to undertake short refresher detoxes on a regular basis; for example, one day each week or fortnight, or a weekend each month. If you have already followed the 30-Day Makeover or Detox in Nine Days programme, you are unlikely to experience any side effects or withdrawal symptoms (see pp. 82–85) during a short refresher detox. If your first detox was shorter, you may notice some unpleasant symptoms, but they usually become milder each time you detox, and eventually they disappear altogether.

For one-day programmes you can choose a mono-diet (see pp. 70–72) or mini-fast (see pp. 70–73). For a weekend try the Weekend Energizer, or the Optional Intensive Plan on p. 48 for a one-day fast combined with one day of light eating. If you started with one of the shorter programmes you can always take your detox experience further by refreshing with the 30-Day Makeover or Detox in Nine Days. Perhaps the ultimate refresher detox programme is to have an annual plan, such as detoxing with the seasons (see box).

DETOX WITH THE **SEASONS**

- Spring provides an ideal time to shake off the winter blues and to follow the 30-Day Makeover. If your are taking a holiday at home, you may prefer the shorter, stricter Detox in Nine Days programme. Either plan will help you to shed any extra pounds that have crept on during the winter months, and prepare you to make the most of the summer ahead.

- Summer brings the new season's vegetables: juice them for an invigorating Weekend Energizer. Alternatively, you may choose to feast on the new season's fruit by following the suggestions for the first two days of the Detox in Nine Days programme.

- Autumn brings cooler weather. Have a mono-diet day with hot cooked food, and add warming spices such as ginger or cinnamon to your hot drinks. Curl up with a book or some music and relax.

- Winter is not a time to fast as you need plenty of good nourishment to help your immune system to fight off 'flu, coughs and colds. Your detox refresher could include a weekend, or a week, on week 2 of the 30-Day Makeover programme (see pp. 52–53). This allows you to eat as much healthy food as you wish, and you can keep the cold at bay by relaxing in a warm bath, perfumed with your favourite aromatherapy oil.

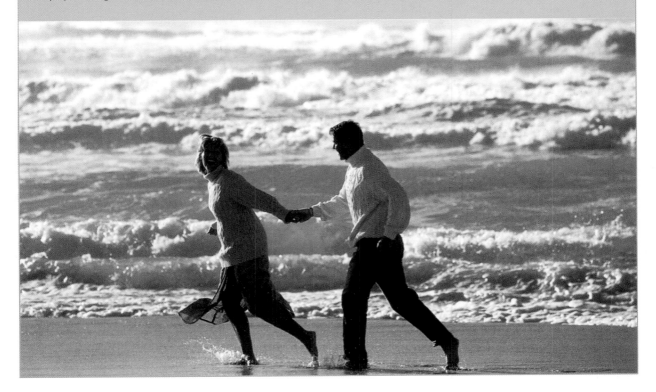

Bodywork **maintenance**

Aerobic exercise (p. 91) brings many health benefits and yoga (pp. 92–93) keeps you supple and calm. Having started these during your detox, why not continue to practise them or look for types of exercise that you find more enjoyable?

To avoid injuring your muscles, remember to warm up for exercise by stretching (see p. 90), and to avoid heaviness and stiffness in your muscles, slow down for a few minutes before stopping. If you are over 30, or have any health problems, including being overweight, discuss your exercise programme with your doctor before you start. Possible ways to exercise include:

Walking and cycling: Gradually build up to exercise for 30–45 minutes, up to five times a week. Wear a mask if you are in a polluted area.

Swimming: Gradually work up to swimming nonstop for 20–40 minutes.

Joining a gym: If you are a beginner find an instructor to help you increase the amount of exercise at a pace that will not cause injury.

Other options: Find a local class or personal teacher for your chosen exercise, such as aerobics, Tai chi, Pilates or yoga. If you prefer a competitive sport join a local team that plays your favourite game, or take up golf.

OTHER BODYWORK AIDS

As part of your lo-tox lifestyle, you may find that continuing to make time for hydrotherapy and skin brushing (see p. 94) will be beneficial. If you find the hydrotherapy suggestions in this book helpful, you could experiment with other forms of hydrotherapy. A consultation with a naturopath may be useful, or you can find out more from a book (see further reading p. 124).

MAINTAINING YOUR CALM

Try to make time to continue with daily meditation (see pp. 102–103). When practised regularly, meditation can help you to stay calm and relaxed, and also improve your efficiency at work. Making time for a regular self-massage (see p. 67) or having a regular aromatherapy massage by a professional are good ongoing aids to mental detox.

EATING WELL

Hippocrates is credited with being the father of medicine. He may have lacked modern equipment and diagnostic aids, but he set down some basic principles that remain relevant today. One of these is his frequently quoted suggestion to 'Let your food be your medicine'.

A healthy diet is an essential part of your maintenance plan, as it limits the amount of unfriendly chemicals your detox system has to cope with. Perhaps more importantly, it provides

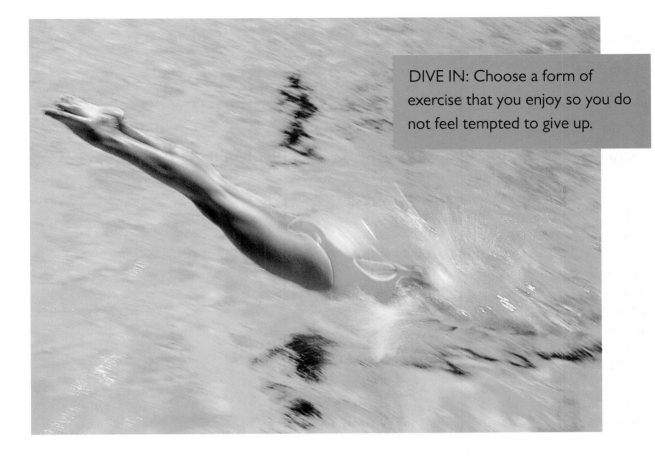

DIVE IN: Choose a form of exercise that you enjoy so you do not feel tempted to give up.

nutrients to fuel your body's detox system, maximize its efficiency and minimize the chances of rebuilding a backlog of toxins. You will find more information about nutrients on the next few pages, but try to avoid junk food and build your diet around the following daily guidelines:

- Six to eight glasses of water (see p. 20). You will need more in hot weather or if you are sweating from exercise or hydrotherapy.
- Two to four servings of fruit and three to five servings of vegetables: a single serving is 75–125g/ 3–4oz. Be sure to include those rich in carotenoids and vitamin C (see p. 44). You can choose to have some of these as juice (see p. 69), but this does remove much of the valuable fibre (see p. 116).
- A modest amount of protein (see pp. 118–119), some fat (see pp. 120–121) and enough whole grain cereals to fill you up (see p. 119). Biscuits, chocolate and cakes often contain hidden fat and sugar.
- Try to restrict alcohol and caffeine to the amounts suggested on pp. 39 and 35. Refined sugar (see p. 36) is best avoided: if you need to sweeten food, use dark brown sugar, molasses, apple juice or sweet fruit such as dates, as these all contain some minerals (see pp. 122–123).

Good value **food**

A nutritionally sound diet contains a good balance of carbohydrates, proteins and fats, sufficient fibre and a plentiful supply of minerals and vitamins. From the detox viewpoint, the best diet will contain as few unfriendly chemicals as possible.

Fibre

Fibre comes from the cell walls and other parts of plants that are not digested. It helps to keep you feeling full for longer after a meal and aids your detox by combining with toxins discharged in the bile so that they are discharged in the stool. Fibre slows the digestive process and helps to regulate the release of glucose into the blood stream. Insufficient fibre appears to contribute to the development of many diseases, including heart disease, gallstones, diabetes, arthritis, certain cancers, diseases of the colon and obesity.

Soluble fibre, which is present in apples, carrots and oats, helps to reduce cholesterol and to balance sugar levels in the blood. Insoluble fibre, found in whole wheat, corn and brown rice, increases the bulk of the stool, reducing the risk of constipation. If you tend to become constipated, it is best not to take wheat bran, which is thought to prevent the absorption of vital vitamins and minerals. Psyllium or linseeds are useful alternatives.

HOW MUCH FIBRE IS NEEDED?

In the United Kingdom, a daily intake of 18g/⅔oz is recommended. In the United States, the Food and Nutrition Board has recommended an increase on the 12g/½oz a day currently eaten by adults.

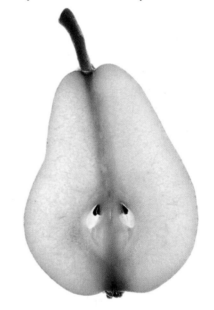

FIBRE CONTENT OF **FOODS**	
Food	Grams of fibre per 100g/3½oz)
Fruits	2–4
Berries	7–9
Nuts	8–14
Cooked beans	5–7
Vegetables	1–2
Wholemeal bread	7

Carbohydrates

Carbohydrates give you energy in the form of sugar. They are present in food as various types of sugars and starch which are digested and absorbed at different rates.

Glucose (dextrose) and sucrose (the sugar in your bowl) are absorbed quickly. They should be eaten sparingly as they can stress the body's ability to maintain a steady level of sugar in the blood (see p. 36). They also appear to depress the immune system. By contrast, the sugar found in most types of fruit, fructose, is absorbed slowly and often incompletely. Starches are simply long chains of sugar molecules, but these have to be broken down into sugar during digestion and are also absorbed more slowly, especially if they are eaten as whole foods. They continue to contribute to the level of sugar in the blood for several hours after a meal.

HOW MUCH IS ENOUGH?

About two-thirds of what you eat should consist of food that is rich in carbs. Many of these, such as fruit, vegetables and milk, also contain a high proportion of water, so the carbs are not densely packed. Only about a fifth of your carbs should come from foods in which the carbs are densely packed, such as grains and dried fruit, or which release their sugar rapidly (see table).

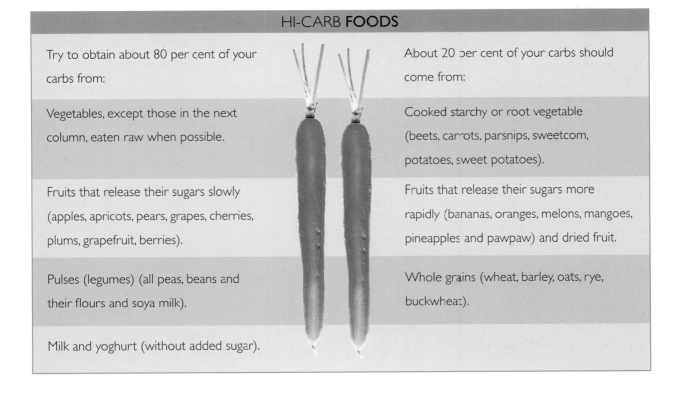

HI-CARB **FOODS**	
Try to obtain about 80 per cent of your carbs from:	About 20 per cent of your carbs should come from:
Vegetables, except those in the next column, eaten raw when possible.	Cooked starchy or root vegetable (beets, carrots, parsnips, sweetcorn, potatoes, sweet potatoes).
Fruits that release their sugars slowly (apples, apricots, pears, grapes, cherries, plums, grapefruit, berries).	Fruits that release their sugars more rapidly (bananas, oranges, melons, mangoes, pineapples and pawpaw) and dried fruit.
Pulses (legumes) (all peas, beans and their flours and soya milk).	Whole grains (wheat, barley, oats, rye, buckwheat).
Milk and yoghurt (without added sugar).	

PROTEINS: Nuts and rice are an excellent source of protein in your diet.

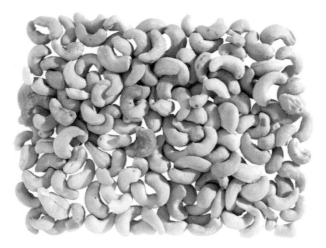

Proteins

Protein is an essential part of every healthy diet. Unlike carbohydrates and fats, you should eat some every day, except for brief periods of fasting, as the building blocks of protein, the amino acids, cannot be stored in your body. Once you have stopped growing, your need for protein is fairly limited, except during pregnancy and lactation. In Western countries protein deficiency is extremely unlikely. Most of the amino acids needed for various functions can be made from other amino acids within your body, but there are a few that have to be obtained from the diet. These are often called 'essential' amino acids.

The amounts of these essential amino acids present in different foods can vary widely. For this reason you should eat protein from a number of different sources in order to obtain enough of each essential amino acid.

Even animal sources of protein do not always contain amino acids in the best possible proportions, and non-vegetarians are well advised to eat vegetable protein, especially cereal proteins, in addition to meat, fish and eggs. Cereals contain an amino acid, methionine, which can be relatively low in animal and other plant proteins; methionine is extremely important for the liver's detox and other functions.

Vegetarians who eat no animal produce at all should ensure that they eat at least two different types of vegetable protein each day (see box), preferably at every meal. Most vegetable proteins are deficient in at least one of the essential amino acids. Exceptions are soya beans and derivatives such as tofu, quinoa, millet and mycoprotein (manufactured commercially as quorn). However, the advice to eat protein from more than one source still applies even if you eat these foods.

PROTEIN AND DETOX

The protein foods that have been suggested in the detox programmes in this book are ones that have received as little processing as possible, and you should continue to eat these foods for your lo-tox maintenance programme. This means that smoked foods such as meat, fish, tofu or cheese, cured meats such as bacon, and foods that are high in fat or contain preservative chemicals such as most sausages, should only be eaten occasionally. Try to buy meat and fish that is still recognizable as part of the original animal, rather than those that have been processed, as this may introduce unknown ingredients and little of the original animal may remain.

HOW MUCH PROTEIN DO WE NEED?

Strange as it may seem, the answer to this question is not known with certainty. Much of the research that has been undertaken has been directed towards avoiding protein deficiency, rather than finding out what is really the healthiest possible intake. At the moment, scientists recommend that you should eat 0.25g of protein each day for each kilogram of your body weight (just under 0.5g per 450g/1lb of body weight). As the effects of eating excess protein are unknown, you are currently advised not to eat more than twice this amount.

VEGETABLE SOURCES OF **PROTEIN**

Wholegrain cereals, e.g. wheat oats and barley.

Nuts, e.g. almonds, pecans and cashews.

Pulses (legumes), e.g. beans, peas and lentils.

Seeds, e.g. pumpkin, sunflower and sesame.

A GUIDE TO **PROTEIN** IN FOOD

Each of these portions contains about 12g/½oz of protein:

60g/2oz lean meat

60g/2oz fish

45g/1½oz Cheddar cheese

100g/3½oz egg

400ml/14fl oz skimmed milk

100g/3½oz oatmeal (uncooked)

100g/3½oz puffed wheat

130g/4½oz wholemeal bread

60g/2oz peanuts

100g/3½oz walnuts

100g/3½oz Brazil nuts

60g/2oz sunflower seeds

60g/2oz tofu (can vary: check manufacturer's figure)

170g/6oz red kidney beans (cooked)

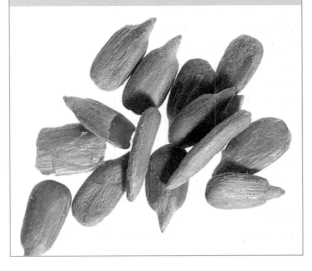

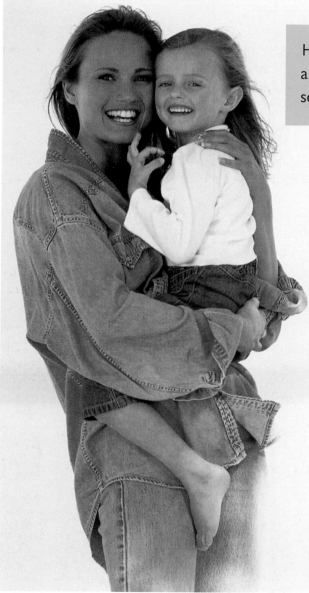

HELP YOUR BRAIN: Eat oily fish twice a week, and small amounts of nuts and seeds on a regular basis.

nervous system, including the brain, to function properly, and for fat-soluble vitamins in the diet to be absorbed. Unfortunately, fat is also high in calories and can be stored easily in the body, sometimes in the walls of arteries which may then become blocked. The amount of fat that you eat has to be limited in order to reduce the risk of heart disease and to avoid putting on weight.

There are various types of fat: saturated fats that are usually solid at room temperature, and unsaturated fats that are usually soft at room temperature and are often called oils. It is the saturated fats that can be most hazardous to health, so you should aim to eat them sparingly.

The unsaturated fats are sometimes called the 'good fats', and there are two types: the monounsaturated fats and the polyunsaturated fats. Monounsaturated fats appear to provide some protection against heart disease, and are the best to use for cooking, as they do not tend to undergo chemical changes when they are heated.

Polyunsaturated fats are prone to undergo chemical changes when they are exposed to light, heat, the air and other chemicals. When they are processed, such as in the manufacture of margarine, chemical changes can occur, leading to the production of 'trans-fats' that the body cannot easily breakdown and which can result in blocked arteries and heart disease.

Fats

In recent years fat has had a bad press. This has not been entirely justified, because fat is an essential part of a healthy diet. Fat is present in the walls of every cell, keeps the skin waterproof and is vital for the

ESSENTIAL FATS

Some types of polyunsaturated fat are known as 'essential', as they have to be eaten in the diet because they cannot be made in our bodies. These come mainly from the omega-6 family of fats and a smaller, but essential, amount from the omega-3 family of fats. Scientists increasingly believe that a balance between them is vital, and that this balance has been disturbed by modern methods of rearing meat and by food processing, in which the less common omega-3 fats are removed because they easily become rancid. The omega-6 fats are widely available in modern diets.

ESSENTIAL FATS AND DETOX

Essential fats play a vital supportive role in detox by helping your immune system, preventing food cravings, keeping the level of sugar steady in the blood, combating fatigue and maintaining steady energy levels. In addition, essential fats help to keep your skin soft and youthful, combat depression and may reduce the risk of developing cancer.

WHAT SORT OF FATS ARE YOU EATING?

Fatty foods contain a mixture of different types of fat. The table below lists the major types of fat in some common foods. Where two types of fat are present in large proportions in a particular food, it appears in more than one list.

HOW MUCH FAT IS ENOUGH?

About 25–30 per cent of calories is probably the optimum fat intake. If you eat 2000 calories a day, this means eating about 60–70g/2–2½oz of fat each day. You can maintain a good intake of omega-3 fats by eating oily fish once or twice a week and/or using cold pressed linseed (flaxseed) or rapeseed (canola) oil. The latter can be mixed into an equal weight of butter to provide a soft spread that is free of trans-fats.

WHAT SORT OF FATS ARE YOU EATING?			
Saturated fats	Monounsaturated fats	Polyunsaturated fats	
		Omega-3 fats	Omega-6 fats
Butter	Olive oil	Fish oil	Corn oil
Red meat fat	Rapeseed (canola) oil	Flaxseed (linseed) oil	Safflower oil
Palm oil	Avocado oil	Rapeseed (canola) oil	Cottonseed oil
Coconut oil	Peanut oil	Walnut oil	Soybean oil
Cocoa butter		Soybean oil	Peanut oil
			Sesame oil
			Grapeseed oil
			Borage oil
			Evening primrose oil

Vitamins and minerals

Vitamins and minerals are known as micro-nutrients, as they are needed in small amounts, but they are absolutely essential to the efficiency of the biochemical processes in the body.

VITAMINS

VITAMIN A (RETINOL AND BETA-CAROTENE)
Found in: fish liver oil, liver, egg yolk, milk, and as beta-carotene in yellow and orange vegetables and fruit.
Needed for: healthy eyes (including night vision), resistance to infection.

VITAMIN B1 (THIAMINE)
Found in: whole grains and whole-grain products, sunflower seeds, seafood, beans.
Needed for: a healthy nervous system, fertility.

VITAMIN B2 (RIBOFLAVIN)
Found in: liver, cheese, eggs, almonds, green leafy vegetables.
Needed for: healthy hair, skin and nails, good eyesight.

VITAMIN B3 (NIACIN)
Found in: nuts, eggs, milk, liver, soy flour, peanut butter, potatoes, avocados.
Needed for: healthy skin and digestive tract, hormone production.

VITAMIN B5 (PANTHOTHENIC ACID)
Found in: nuts, wheat germ, pulses (legumes), eggs, green vegetables.
Needed for: hormone production, healthy skin, muscles and nerves.

VITAMIN B6 (PYRIDOXINE)
Found in: offal, sunflower seeds, wheatgerm, beans, eggs, liver.
Needed for: healthy immune system, balancing hormone changes in women.

VITAMIN B12
Found in: liver, oily fish, egg yolks.
Needed for: to prevent anaemia, infection, mental deterioration in old age.

VITAMIN C
Found in: fresh fruit and vegetablis.
Needed for: to combat infection, poor wound healing, heart disease.

VITAMIN D (CALCIFEROL)

Found in: fish liver oils, green leafy vegetables, mushrooms, eggs, milk, butter.

Needed for: healthy heart and nervous system.

VITAMIN E (TOCOPHEROL)

Found in: wheat germ oil, nuts, seeds, whole grains.

Needed for: healthy cell membranes, fertility, stamina, combating changes of old age.

FOLIC ACID

Found in: leafy green vegetables, fruit, whole grains, liver, milk.

Needed for: prevention of anaemia, heart disease, congenital abnormalities.

VITAMIN K

Found in: leafy vegetables, cheese, liver.

Needed for: blood clotting, healthy bones and teeth.

MINERALS

CALCIUM

Found in: hard water, milk, cheese, green leafy vegetables, seeds, nuts.

Needed for: healthy bones, teeth and muscles.

CHROMIUM

Found in: egg yolk, molasses, red meat, wine, whole grains, vegetables.

Needed for: maintenance of correct blood sugar levels and cholesterol.

COPPER

Found in: seafood, pulses (legumes) olives, nuts.

Needed for: blood, bones and nervous system.

IODINE

Found in: fish, sea vegetables.

Needed for: thyroid gland to function effectively.

IRON

Found in: liver, red meat, whole grains, pulses (legumes), green vegetables.

Needed for: to prevent anaemia.

MAGNESIUM

Found in: nuts, whole grains, fruit, green vegetables, hard water.

Needed for: normal muscle function and blood pressure, to prevent fatigue.

POTASSIUM

Found in: fruit, vegetables, salmon, lamb.

Needed for: healthy bones, to combat fatigue and muscle weakness.

SELENIUM

Found in: Brazil nuts, seafood, whole grains, eggs.

Needed for: to fight infection, for detox.

SODIUM

Found in: salt and salty foods.

Needed for: regulating the water in the body.

ZINC

Found in: seafood, whole grains, nuts, seeds.

Needed for: to fight infection, repair wounds, normal sexual function.

Further **reading**

NUTRITION

Aphrodite Diet, The, Dr Artemis Simopoulos and
Jo Robinson (Published by Vermilion)

Detoxification and Healing, Sidney MacDonald Baker
MD (Published by Keats Publishing Inc.)

Electropollution, Roger Coghill
(Published by Thorsons)

Environmental Medicine in Clinical Practice,
Honor Anthony, Sybil Birtwhistle, Keith Eaton,
Jonathan Maberly (Published by BSAENM
Publications)

Fats that Heal Fats that Kill, Udo Erasmus
(Published by Alive books)

Herb Bible, The, Earl Mindell
(Published by Vermilion)

Hydrotherapy, Leon Chaito
(Published by Element)

Juice and Zest Book, Anna Selby
(Published by Collins & Brown)

Liver Cleansing Diet, The, Sandra Cabot MD
(Published by Women's Health Advisory Service)

Liver Detox Plan, Xandria Williams
(Published by Vermilion)

Potatoes not Prozac, Kathleen DesMaisons
(Published by Simon and Schuster)

Textbook of Natural Medicine, Eds Joseph E. Pizzorno
and Michael T. Murray (Published by Churchill
Livingstone)

20-day Rejuvenation Program, The, Jeffrey Bland
(Published by Keats Publishing Inc.)

Vitamin Alphabet, The, Dr Christina Scott-Moncrieft
(Published by Collins & Brown)

RELATED SUBJECTS

Aroma Remedies, Chrissy Wildwood
(Published by Collins & Brown)

4 Weeks to Total Energy, Judith Wills
(Published by Quadrille Publishing Ltd)

Homeopathy for Women, Barry Rose and Christina
Scott-Moncrieff (Published by Collins & Brown)

Stress Protection Plan, The, Suzannah Olivier
(Published by Collins & Brown)

Yoga for Stress, Vimla Lalvani
(Published by Hamlyn)

Yoga, Mind and Body, Sivananda Vedanta Centre
(Published by Dorling Kindersley)

Useful **addresses**

Herbalism

American Herb Association
P. O. Box 1673
Nevada City
California 95959
USA

American Herbalists Guild
P.O. Box 1683
Sequel
California 95073
USA
Tel: 408 484 244

British Herbal Medicine Association
1 Wickham Road, Boscombe
Bournemouth BH7 6JX
Tel: 01202 433691

National Institute of Medical Herbalists
56 Longbrooke Street
Exeter EX4 8HA
Tel: 01392 426022

Homeopathy
British Homeopathic Association
15 Clerkenwell Close
London ECIR OAA
Tel: 020 7566 7800

National Center for Homeopathy
801 North Fairfax Street
Suite 306
Alexandria
Virginia
USA
Tel: 703 548 7790

Society of Homeopaths
4A Artizan Road
Northampton NNI 4HU
Tel: 01604 621400

Nutrition

American Association of World Health
1129–2012 st, NW, ste. 400
Washington DC 20036 34 03
USA

British Nutritional Foundation
52–54 High Holborn
London WCIV 6RQ
Tel: 020 7404 6504

Institute for Optimum Nutrition
Blade's Court
Deodar Road
London SW15 2NU
Tel: 020 8877 9993

National Institute of Nutritional Education
1010 S. Jolier St, Aurora,
CO 80012
USA
Tel: 303 340 2054

Society for the Promotion of Nutritional Therapy
P.O. Box 626
Woking GU22 OXD
Tel: 01483 740903

Yoga

British Wheel of Yoga
1 Hamilton Place, Boston Road
Sleaford Lines NG34 7ES
Tel: 01529 306851

Yoga for Health Foundation
Ickwell Bury, Ickwell Green
Nr Biggleswade
Bedfordshire SG 18 9EF
Tel: 01767 627271

Yoga ResearchCenter
P.O. Box 1386, Lower Lake
California 95457
USA
Tel: 707 928 9898

Index

Acknowledgements

Photographs are copyright © as follows:

Jacket (front left) Don Lowe/Gettyone Stone
Jacket (front right) Powerstock Zefa
Page 3 Charles Thatcher/Gettyone Stone
Page 7 The Photographers Library
Page 11 (top left) Jeremy Walker/Science Photo Library
Page 11 (top right) Mike McQueen/Gettyone Stone
Page 13 Megumi Miyatake/Telegraph Colour Library
Page 15 Antonio Mo/Telegraph Colour Library
Page 17 The Photographers Library
Page 19 The Photographers Library
Page 21 John Slater/Telegraph Colour Library
Page 24 Powerstock Zefa
Page 25 The Photographers Library
Page 26 Powerstock Zefa
Page 31 Michelangelo Gratton/Gettyone Stone
Page 33 Stuart McClymont/Gettyone Stone
Page 34 Beth Ava/Telegraph Colour Library
Page 35 Powerstock Zefa
Page 37 Powerstock Zefa
Page 38 Paul Viant/Telegraph Colour Library
Page 40 Richard Laird/Telegraph Colour Library
Page 43 Powerstock Zefa
Page 48 James Darell/Gettyone Stone
Page 51 Chris Harvey/Gettyone Stone
Page 53 James Darell/Gettyone Stone
Page 54 Chris Craymer/Gettyone Stone
Page 57 Dennis O'Clair/Gettyone Stone
Page 58 J.P. Fruchet/Telegraph Colour Library
Page 62 The Photographers Library
Page 65 Neo Vision/Photonica
Page 67 Paul Viant/Telegraph Colour Library
Page 76 James Darell/Gettyone Stone
Page 80 Dennis O'Clair/Gettyone Stone
Page 81 The Photographers Library

Page 82 Dale Durtee/Gettyone Stone
Page 84 The Photographers Library
Page 86 Powerstock Zefa
Page 89 The Photographers Library
Page 90 Powerstock Zefa
Page 91 J.P. Lefret/Telegraph Colour Library
Page 92 The Photographers Library
Page 95 Chris Craymer/Gettyone Stone
Page 96 Gettyone Stone
Page 97 (right) Peter Nicholson/Gettyone Stone
Page 98 Powerstock Zefa
Page 99 The Photographers Library
Page 101 Chris Craymer/Gettyone Stone
Page 103 Anthony Marsland/Gettyone Stone
Page 107 The Photographers Library
Page 113 Powerstock Zefa
Page 115 Powerstock Zefa
Page 120 The Photographers Library

All other photographs are copyright ©
Collins & Brown.

Dr Christina Scott-Moncrieff is a doctor, homeopathic physician and a member of the British Society for Allergy, Environmental and Nutritional Medicine. She is the best-selling author of:
THE VITAMIN ALPHABET
Dr Christina Scott-Moncrieff (1 85585 681 6)
HOMEOPATHY FOR WOMEN
Dr Barry Rose & Dr Christina Scott-Moncrieff
(1 85028 392 3)
NATURAL HEALTH AT 50+
Dr Christina Scott-Moncrieff (1 85585 777 4)